PHARMACOLOGY - RESEARCH, SAFETY TESTING AND REGULATION

DRY POWDER INHALERS

FORMULATION, DEVICE AND CHARACTERIZATION

PHARMACOLOGY - RESEARCH, SAFETY TESTING AND REGULATION

Additional books in this series can be found on Nova's website
under the Series tab.

Additional e-books in this series can be found on Nova's website
under the eBook tab.

PHARMACOLOGY - RESEARCH, SAFETY TESTING AND REGULATION

DRY POWDER INHALERS

FORMULATION, DEVICE AND CHARACTERIZATION

TEERAPOL SRICHANA

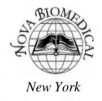

New York

NOTICE TO THE READER

Library of Congress Cataloging-in-Publication Data

ISBN: 978-1-53610-641-1

Library of Congress Control Number: 2016960251

Published by Nova Science Publishers, Inc. † *New York*

Contents

Preface

This book is a compilation of most works published during 2000-2016 in the area of dry powder inhalers, especially related to the issues with formulation and device design. The dry powder inhalers aim to deliver the medication to the respiratory airways. It is suitable for postgraduate students and researchers who work in the areas of dry powder inhalers. It provides some background knowledge in size characterization, flow properties, forces, and interaction of air and particles. It also ends with *in vitro* quality control of dry powder inhalers. This book was finished in Hawaii where the author spent his time during April 2016. Thank you to Prince of Songkla University for the financial support. The author had to work very hard for one month without a holiday. Thank you to Prof. Aran Pattanothai for overseeing this work to make sure that the researchers were on schedule all the time. Thanks to the author's staff at the Graduate School, Prince of Songkla University who had to work hard and be patient when the author was not in the office. Thanks to the author's wife and son who had to wait for him at home in Thailand. Thanks to Dr. Tan Suwandecha and Dr. Janwit Dechraksa for their great efforts in copy editing and compiling all the references. The author also thanks Dr. Somchai Sawatdee and Dr. Dhamodharan Bakkiyaraj for their comments, and Dr. Padmavathi Alwar Ramanujam for her proofreading. The greatest help was from Professor Alan Coombes, Professor Pornanong Aramwit, and Dr. Brian Hodgeson for their criticisms and comments to make this book readable.

Teerapol Srichana, Ph.D.
Prince of Songkla University
Hat Yai, Thailand

General Introduction

Why Dry Powder Inhalers?

The lungs are an attractive route to deliver therapeutics for both local and systemic therapy. A drug delivery system as an aerosol offers additional degrees of manipulation to target the organ and specific cells. Pulmonary delivery systems have many challenges including poor delivery efficiency, instability of drugs and their formulations, and poor uniformity. Nevertheless, these systems offer many advantages over oral routes such as higher bioavailability and lower dose and less invasiveness in comparison with injectable dosage forms. The lungs have a large surface area for absorption and limited proteolytic enzymes. Together with its thin epithelial layer, it gives high drug permeability and drugs can be delivered specifically to the target areas. A targeted delivery system can reduce the dose and side effects from low systemic exposure.

Not only is the local drug delivered to the target organ but also systemic drug delivery can be done by targeting the alveolar regions (Patton and Byron 2007). A systemic delivery system can achieve a rapid onset and avoid first pass metabolism. It is also useful for the delivery of biotherapeutics that cannot be delivered orally. Furthermore, for the treatment of lung tuberculosis, the therapeutics can be targeted to specific lung cells such as alveolar macrophages (Changsan, Nilkaeo, et al. 2009).

The lungs can be exposed to various materials from different sources in the breathing process. These airborne particles deposit along the airways from the oropharynx, trachea, bronchi, bronchioles down to the respiratory bronchioles and alveolar sacs. Particles are rapidly cleared by cilia within the mucus layer in the upper airways and by mucociliary escalator in the lower airways. The pulmonary epithelium acts as a barrier to absorption in the airways. The epithelium of the lung diminishes towards the lower airways to a thickness of 0.2 μm in the alveoli. Gas exchange occurs in the alveolar region. The vast surface area of the alveoli with high blood supply from the capillary arteries provides a great access of therapeutics to a systemic circulation. The airways are protected by immune cells especially alveolar macrophages to scavenge foreign materials along the lung surface (Fels and Cohn 1986).

Particles entering the lung are deposited along the airways by inertial impaction, sedimentation, and diffusion (Hinds 2012). These particles are characterized by their aerodynamic diameter. Large particles (> 5 μm) are deposited by inertial impaction in the mouth and upper airways, whereas the smaller particles are deposited deeper in the lungs. Very small particles are driven by diffusion.

Several technologies exist to deliver therapeutics to the airways. Nebulizers have been used for a long time to deliver mists of a drug by ultrasonic or air-jet mechanism. However, these devices tend to limit their usage only at hospitals or home. Significant advances in medical aerosol technology began in early 1950 with a focus on delivering asthmatic drugs directly to the lungs thereby significantly reducing the dose and thus limiting side effects. The first product was a handheld delivery system, a metered dose inhaler (MDI), where the drugs were suspended in the compressed liquid gas. However, these devices varied in particle deposition in the lungs depending on the device, formulation and inspiratory effort of the patient. Alternatives were then introduced as dry powder inhalers (DPI).

History of the Dry Powder Inhaler

DPI was established nearly 50 years after the MDI. Since the DPI is in a solid state, it is suitable for unstable drugs in a liquid dosage form, and it does not need a propellant gas. However, the MDI is commonly prescribed at the first visit of an asthmatic or chronic obstructive pulmonary disease patient. Later on, if the patient finds it difficult to comply with the MDI, the patient may ask the doctor to change the prescription. Today, it is easy to switch from the MDI to the DPI as several pharmaceutical manufacturers produce both types of inhalers as a choice for the patients. The first DPI utilized the patient's inspiratory effort to disperse micronized drug particles. Further development has focused on the device development and particle engineering. Compressed air may be supplied from the advanced device. Different sizes and shapes of particles are designed to deposit in the alveolar regions.

Dry Powder Inhaler Formulation

DPI formulations are usually prepared as homogeneous interactive mixtures comprised of micronized drug particles and a coarse carrier (Malcolmson and Embleton 1998). The coarse carrier employed in the DPI formulation is commonly α-lactose monohydrate to improve flow properties and dose uniformity of highly cohesive drug particles. The entrainment and subsequent aerosolization of the formulation are achieved using patient inspiratory effort which is required to elutriate the micronized drug from the carrier surface.

A critical step in generating a therapeutic aerosol via the DPI device is the fluidization and entrainment of the bulk powder. Powder fluidization is a process by which the powder mass is disturbed by a stream of airflow resulting in the powder bed exhibiting fluid-like properties.

To achieve the goal of delivering drugs to the lung region, it is accepted that particles must have an aerodynamic size of 1-5 μm (Hickey 2004). However, particles of this size will have a high surface free energy and therefore have a tendency to adhere together or to any other surface that they might encounter to reduce this surface energy. Therefore, the knowledge of particles, particle–particle interactions, and flow properties are essential for the production of effective DPIs. The interaction between micronized drugs and carrier particles has received much attention. Hence the number of previous studies on this subject is high. In this book, only a few aspects related to the performance of the powder formulations of the DPIs are discussed. The adhesion forces between the carrier particles and drug particles consist mainly of van der Waals forces, electrostatic forces and capillary forces. Van der Waals forces are the most dominant forces that can determine adhesion or cohesion in powders that are inhaled. Compared with electrostatic and capillary forces, van der Waals forces are lower, which is a desirable property from the viewpoint of dispersion during inhalation. Moreover, they can be controlled to a certain extent and are more constant over longer periods.

The research areas that involve adhesive mixtures for inhalation have explored the control of the properties of the carrier surface and measuring the adhesive forces between the drug and carrier using centrifugal techniques and atomic force microscopy. Mixing theories have been developed based on the assumption that competition exists during mixing between drug–drug and drug–carrier interactions and the equilibrium between them that occurs at any moment during the mixing process. It has also been postulated that the equilibrium can be driven in a certain direction by modifying the carrier surface properties. Much attention has been given to the so-called 'active sites' on the carrier surface, onto which the drug particles are attached to higher adhesive forces than the other sites. The term 'active site' has been used for a multitude of phenomena including surface irregularities, surface rugosity and adhering fines. Several investigations have attempted to modify and control the surface rugosity of carrier crystals. The effects of carrier payloads, mixing conditions, drug-to-carrier interactions, and the type and magnitude of the removal forces during inhalation have been reported. Lactose monohydrate is one of the most common carrier materials used in the DPI formulations. Other sugars such as glucose and mannitol are also acceptable. In addition, biodegradable polymers, phospholipids, cholesterol derivatives, cholates and amino acids have been studied (Chuealee, Aramwit, and Srichana 2007, Changsan, Nilkaeo, et al. 2009, Changsan, Chan, et al. 2009, Chuealee, Wiedmann, and Srichana 2009, Chuealee et al. 2010, Rojanarat et al. 2011, Chuealee, Wiedmann, and Srichana 2011, Rojanarat et al. 2012, Rattanupatam and Srichana 2014, Gangadhar, Adhikari, and Srichana 2014, Ahmad, Nakpheng, and Srichana 2014, Ahmad, Ungphaiboon, and Srichana 2015, Kaewjan and Srichana 2016). Mixtures of lactose with the drug are often called interactive mixtures, which are easier to handle during the manufacturing process than micronized drugs. The use of a carrier also makes the handling of small drug doses possible. The drug particles should loosely adhere to the carrier particles so that they will easily detach from the carrier particles and become available for deposition in the lungs. The larger carriers impact tissues in the mouth or at the back of the throat and are swallowed. The carrier also provides bulk to the formulation, which improves the handling, dispensing and metering of the drug dose, which is of particular importance for low dose formulations. To ensure efficient drug delivery, it is critical that adhesive forces between the drug and carrier are not too strong. Otherwise, the detachment of the drug from the carrier will be difficult or not possible. Hence, the balance between adhesive and cohesive forces should be adjusted to ensure sufficient adhesion between the drug and carrier to provide a homogeneous blend with a uniform content. It is recognized that the efficiency of a powder formulation is highly dependent on the carrier, the particle size and size distribution, the inhalation flow rate, and the dispersion efficiency of the respective DPI device.

Three different formulation types exist: spherical pellets, adhesive mixtures, and particle agglomerates. In general, the micronized drug is formulated into a powder mixture to improve dose uniformity and filling process. Drug particles should be distributed homogeneously over the total surface area of the carrier and should attach to the carrier surface primarily by van der Waals forces. Carriers in adhesive mixtures consist of appropriate size fractions. When the drug is distributed in multi-particulate layers around carrier particles, agglomerates are formed. Carrier size distribution must then be selected to obtain good flow properties, which is a prerequisite for reproducible measurements of the dose.

The DPI platform is characterized by dispensing the medication to the patient as a dry powder using a device specifically designed for that formulation. In general, the inhalers employ the patient's inspiratory flow as a means to disperse and transport the aerosols into the lungs. Therefore we usually call them breath-actuated devices. However, nowadays active devices have been made where the device itself produces the aerosol while disregarding the patient's effort.

Dry Powder Inhaler Device

As for the design of the inhaler, this is one of the most important technical aspects to be taken into account when designing and evaluating DPIs. There must be a particular emphasis on the principles of powder de-agglomeration and the moment at which the drug in the aerosol is released (Kwok and Chan 2011). The airflow is generated by the patient through the inhaler especially for breath-actuated devices resulting in fluid and particle dynamics.

Considering the powder de-agglomeration efficiency, the drug particles in dry powder formulations cannot be released as primary entities (1-2 µm) from the DPI. By slightly increasing the primary drug particle size, even within this narrow range, the detached mass fraction of the drug can be increased substantially, particularly for inhalers with poor de-agglomeration efficiency.

The de-agglomeration system of the inhaler is one of the most important steps that determines deposition of the drug in the lung. The de-agglomeration system should break-up the spherical pellets into primary drug particles or detach the drug particles from the carrier in the mixtures or agglomerates during inhalation. The adhesive forces between the drug and carrier particles or the cohesive forces between drug particles have to be aerosolized to primary drug particles. Different de-agglomeration systems use a different mechanism to generate the aerosols. Clearly, the more efficient the force, the higher fine particle fraction (FPF). Powder de-agglomeration systems in DPIs vary considerably by their principle of operation. Most DPIs are often breath-activated systems that utilize the kinetic energy of the inspiratory flow. The sources of auxiliary energy are electromechanical means and pressurized air. The efficacy of detachment of the drug particle will increase with an increase in the inspiratory flow rate through the inhaler. This effect is most pronounced when the kinetic energy of the air flow is utilized more efficiently. In contrast, battery- and pressurized air-operated DPIs performance is not dependent on the inhalation process. However, they are much more complex in design and expensive. These devices may be inappropriate for use as disposable devices.

The performance of the inhaler obviously relies on many aspects including the design of the inhaler, the device resistance, the de-agglomeration systems, the formulation and the inspiratory air flow.

Well-designed DPIs are highly efficient systems, but they are also complicated. The ideal DPI system should include most or all of the following attributes (EMEA 2006): simple and comfortable to use; compact and economical to produce; a stable multiple dose system; a reproducible emitted dose over a wide range of inspiratory flow rates that are consistent and stable throughout the inhalers life span; allow for highly reproducible fine particle dosing; an ability to produce a physically and chemically stable powder; a minimal extrapulmonary loss of the drug (low oropharyngeal deposition, low device retention and low exhaled loss); protection of the powder from the external environment and be usable in all climates; protection against overdose and a dose delivery indicator; suitability for a wide range of drugs and doses.

DPIs can be single or multi-dose (multiple unit doses and multiple doses), depending on the design of the powder reservoir and metering components. In single dose devices, an individual dose is provided. However, they present a weakness since drug loading is required. DPIs with multiple unit doses contain a number of individually packaged doses, either as multiple gelatin capsules or in blisters. In a multiple dose device, bulk powder reservoirs are in the device from which an individual dose is metered.

The DPI device should help in the generation of very fine particles of the drug in a way that enables them to avoid any impaction with barriers in the lung. This mechanism also prevents the ingress of potentially harmful particles to the airways. Most recently there has been an increasing trend to focus on the optimization of the powder-device technology to improve the generation of the aerosol. In general, the inhaler design, particularly the geometry of the mouthpiece, is critical for patients to produce a sufficient airflow to propel the drug from the capsule or reservoir and break up the agglomerates in a turbulent airstream. This device will then deliver a drug dose to the lungs as therapeutically effective fine particles. Each inhaler will have a device that is resistant to the airflow (measured as the square root of the pressure drop across the device divided by the flow rate through the device). Current designs of DPI devices have specific resistance values that range from about 0.02 to 0.2 (cm $H_2O)^{1/2}$/liter per min (LPM) (Newman and Busse 2002). In order to produce a fine powder aerosol with an increased delivery to the lung, a DPI should have a low resistance which needs an inspiratory flow of 90 LPM, a medium resistance DPI requires 50-60 LPM and a high resistance DPI requires 30-40 LPM (Lavorini 2013).

Production Technology

A multitude of techniques has been applied to improve the performance of dry powder formulations for inhalation as listed below:

- Through the addition of micronized ternary excipients such as isoleucine or magnesium stearate that decrease the adhesive forces between the carrier and drug, mainly because the micronized excipient and the drug compete for the active sites. However, the use of magnesium stearate for inhalation raises questions related to safety.
- Supercritical fluid technology has been applied to improve polymorphic purity and the surface properties of the drug substance that can reduce the adhesive forces between the drug and carrier.
- Large porous particles with a high porosity and low density have been produced for several reasons; the most important are the improved de-agglomeration and aerodynamic size. Besides, they are also of interest from the reduced phagocytosis of the deposited particles in the alveoli. The macrophage uptake does not occur, so this prolongs the release of the drug from the particles in the alveolar region. Smaller porous particles (3-5 μm) have also been used to improve de-agglomeration and lung deposition.

- Spray dried, spray freeze-dried drugs and excipients can be used to incorporate unstable drugs into stabilizing matrices like sugar or polyol.
- New materials such as deoxycholate derivatives, cholesterol derivatives, chitosans and their derivatives, and PLGA have been introduced into dry powder formulations.
- Solid lipid nanoparticles, Trojan microparticles, and dimple-shaped carriers have been introduced.

Many trends in the design and development of inhalation devices and formulations can be seen in the literature. Several DPIs were under development in the year 2000 and more recently even a higher number of inhalers are in the pipeline. These new developments result in significant improvements in DPI therapy. Computer simulations have been introduced to understand the flow properties of the formulations in the inhaler devices. The fluid dynamics and powder de-aggregation have been under investigation for a number of years to understand the mechanism of drug particle releases, which is not possible to visualize in an experiment. This *in silico* technology helps us to understand the mechanism behind this technology.

In vitro quality control is essential for DPIs. This is a concern for the manufacturer to ensure that the inhalation products meet the criteria indicated in the Pharmacopeia. In this book, all the methods and general requirements for *in vitro* tests of dry powders are summarized and grouped for readers with some examples of certificates of analysis and data comparisons among the new DPIs.

Next Generation Dry Powder Inhaler

It can be predicted that new formulations and new device technologies for DPIs will be introduced in the next decade. Also, new biotechnology developments will stimulate the growth of new DPIs. Other factors are the possibility of new emerging respiratory diseases and outbreaks of new viral infections that will also promote study in this area of drug delivery. It is predicted that new DPIs that arise by making use of advancements in technology and capability will solve many current problems associated with the delivery of drugs. However, the technical background of inhalation technology aspects has to be tuned to obtain the desired performance of dry powder inhalers. Possible new advances in technical knowledge, new developments and the possibilities for further improvements have been gathered together and have been discussed in the book.

References

Ahmad, Md Iftekhar, Titpawan Nakpheng, and Teerapol Srichana. 2014. "The safety of ethambutol dihydrochloride dry powder formulations containing chitosan for the possibility of treating lung tuberculosis." *Inhalation Toxicology* 26 (14):908-917.

Ahmad, Md Iftekhar, Suwipa Ungphaiboon, and Teerapol Srichana. 2015. "The development of dimple-shaped chitosan carrier for ethambutol dihydrochloride dry powder inhaler." *Drug Development and Industrial Pharmacy* 41 (5):791-800.

Changsan, Narumon, Hak-Kim Chan, Frances Separovic, and Teerapol Srichana. 2009. "Physicochemical characterization and stability of rifampicin liposome dry powder formulations for inhalation." *Journal of Pharmaceutical Sciences* 98 (2):628-639. doi: 10.1002/jps.21441.

Changsan, Narumon, Athip Nilkaeo, Pethchawan Pungrassami, and Teerapol Srichana. 2009. "Monitoring safety of liposomes containing rifampicin on respiratory cell lines and in vitro efficacy against Mycobacterium bovis in alveolar macrophages." *Journal of Drug Targeting* 17 (10):751-762. doi: 10.3109/10611860903079462.

Chuealee, Rabkwan, Pornanong Aramwit, and Teerapol Srichana. 2007. "Characteristics of cholesteryl cetyl carbonate liquid crystals as drug delivery systems." Proceedings of the 2nd IEEE International Conference on Nano/Micro Engineered and Molecular Systems, IEEE NEMS 2007.

Chuealee, Rabkwan, Timothy Scott Wiedmann, and Teerapol Srichana. 2009. "Thermotropic behavior of sodium cholesteryl carbonate." *Journal of Materials Research* 24 (1):156-163. doi: 10.1557/jmr.2009.0027.

Chuealee, Rabkwan, Timothy Scott Wiedmann, and Teerapol Srichana. 2011. "Physicochemical properties and antifungal activity of amphotericin b incorporated in cholesteryl carbonate esters." *Journal of Pharmaceutical Sciences* 100 (5):1727-1735. doi: 10.1002/jps.22398.

Chuealee, Rabkwan, Timothy Scott Wiedmann, Roongnapa Suedee, and Teerapol Srichana. 2010. "Interaction of Amphotericin B with cholesteryl palmityl carbonate ester." *Journal of Pharmaceutical Sciences* 99 (11):4593-4602. doi: 10.1002/jps.22176.

EMEA. 2006. Guideline on the pharmaceutical quality of inhalation and nasal products.

Fels, Anna O., and Zanvil A. Cohn. 1986. "The alveolar macrophage." *Journal of Applied Physiology* 60 (2):353-369.

Gangadhar, Katkam N., Kajiram Adhikari, and Teerapol Srichana. 2014. "Synthesis and evaluation of sodium deoxycholate sulfate as a lipid drug carrier to enhance the solubility, stability and safety of an amphotericin B inhalation formulation." *International Journal of Pharmaceutics* 471 (1-2):430-438. doi: 10.1016/j.ijpharm.2014.05.066.

Hickey, Anthony J. 2004. "Pharmaceutical Inhalation Aerosol Technology." *American Association of Pharmaceuticals Scientists, 2nd ed Marcel Dekker, Inc: NewYork.*

Hinds, William C. 2012. *Aerosol Technology: Properties, Behavior, and Measurement of Airborne Particles*: John Wiley & Sons.

Kaewjan, Kanogwan, and Teerapol Srichana. 2016. "Nano spray-dried pyrazinamide-l-leucine dry powders, physical properties and feasibility used as dry powder aerosols." *Pharmaceutical Development and Technology* 21 (1):68-75. doi: 10.3109/10837450.2014.971373.

Kwok, Philip CL, and Hak-Kim Chan. 2011. "Pulmonary delivery of peptide and proteins." *Peptide and Protein Delivery, Elsevier Inc., London*: 23-46.

Lavorini, Federico. 2013. "The challenge of delivering therapeutic aerosols to asthma patients." *ISRN Allergy* 2013.

Malcolmson, Richard J, and Jonathan K Embleton. 1998. "Dry powder formulations for pulmonary delivery." *Pharmaceutical Science & Technology Today* 1 (9):394-398.

Newman, Simon P, and William W. Busse. 2002. "Evolution of dry powder inhaler design, formulation, and performance." *Respiratory Medicine* 96 (5):293-304.

Patton, John S., and Peter R. Byron. 2007. "Inhaling medicines: delivering drugs to the body through the lungs." *Nature Reviews Drug Discovery* 6 (1):67-74.

Rattanupatam, Teerarat, and Teerapol Srichana. 2014. "Budesonide dry powder for inhalation: Effects of leucine and mannitol on the efficiency of delivery." *Drug Delivery* 21 (6):397-405. doi: 10.3109/10717544.2013.868555.

Rojanarat, Wipaporn, Narumon Changsan, Ekawat Tawithong, Sirirat Pinsuwan, Hak-Kim Chan, and Teerapol Srichana. 2011. "Isoniazid proliposome powders for inhalation-preparation, characterization and cell culture studies." *International Journal of Molecular Sciences* 12 (7):4414-4434. doi: 10.3390/ijms12074414.

Rojanarat, Wipaporn, Titpawan Nakpheng, Ekawat Thawithong, Niracha Yanyium, and Teerapol Srichana. 2012. "Inhaled pyrazinamide proliposome for targeting alveolar macrophages." *Drug Delivery* 19 (7):334-345. doi: 10.3109/10717544.2012.721144.

Chapter 1

Particle Size and Size Characterization of Aerosols

1.1. Introduction

Aerosols are ubiquitous in our environment. The physical properties of aerosol particles and their determination by scientific means have been developed to predict their behavior. To begin a systematic study of particles, it is necessary to consider several commonly used definitions of aerosols. Aerosols are suspensions of solid or liquid particles in a gas, usually air.

1.2. Morphological Properties of Aerosols

It is convenient to think of all aerosol particles as spheres for calculations, and this also helps to visualize the processes taking place. A particle is generally imagined to be spherical or nearly spherical. Either the particle radius or particle diameter can be used to describe a particle's size. Thus one should ascertain which definition is being used when the term particle size is used. Once a choice of diameter or radius is made, there are a number of ways to define the diameter or radius which reflect particle properties other than physical size. For a monodisperse aerosol, a single measure describes the diameter of all particles. However, with polydisperse aerosols a single diameter is insufficient to describe all particle diameters and certain presumptions need to be made on the distribution of sizes. Other parameters in addition to diameter must be used.

Two commonly encountered definitions of particle size are the Feret's diameter and Martin's diameter (Sinko 2006). These refer to estimating the particle size when determined by viewing the projected images of a number of irregularly shaped particles. Feret's diameter is the maximum distance from the edge to edge of each particle, and Martin's diameter is the length of the line that separates each particle into two equal portions. Since these measures can vary depending on the orientation of the particle, they are valid only if averaged over a number of particles and if all measurements are made parallel to one another. Then, by assuming random orientation of the particles, an average diameter is determined. This measurement problem can be simplified to an extent by using the projected area diameter instead of the Feret's diameter or Martin's diameter. This is defined as the diameter of a circle having the same projected area as the particle in question. Figure 1.1 illustrates these three definitions. In general, the Feret's diameter will be larger than the projected area diameter and the projected area diameter will be larger than the Martin's diameter.

Sometimes a diameter is defined in terms of particle settling velocity. All particles having similar settling velocities are considered to be of similar size, regardless of their actual size or shape (Figure 1.2). Two such definitions are aerodynamic diameter and Stokes' diameter.

The aerodynamic diameter is a diameter of a unit density of sphere having the same aerodynamic properties as the particle in question. This means that particles of any shape or density will have the same aerodynamic diameter if their settling velocity is the same (Hickey 2004).

Stokes' diameter is a diameter of a sphere of the same density as the particle in question having the same settling velocity. Stokes' diameter and aerodynamic diameter differ only in that Stokes' diameter includes the particle density whereas the aerodynamic diameter does not.

Aerosol sizes cover a range of about four orders of magnitude from 0.01 μm as a lower limit to approximately 100 μm as the upper limit. Particles larger than 100 μm do not remain suspended in the air for a sufficient length of time to be much of interest in aerosol science. Particles between 5 to 10 μm are usually removed by the upper airways and those smaller than 5 μm can penetrate deep into the alveoli of the lung. Particle size is the most important descriptor for predicting aerosol behavior (Hickey 2004). This is apparent from the above discussion and will become even more apparent in later chapters.

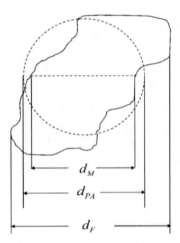

Figure 1.1. Martin's (d_M), projected area (d_{PA}) and Feret's diameter (d_F) for an irregular shaped particle.

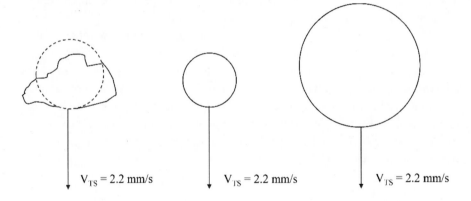

Figure 1.2. Particles with similar setting velocities are equivalent spheres.

1.3. Particle Size Distributions

The first step is to divide the entire size range into a series of successive particle size intervals and determine the number of particles (the count) in each interval. The intervals must be continuous so that no particles are left out. It should have 10 size intervals for 1,000 particles. An example of particle size distribution is shown in Table 1.1. When a particle size is grouped in intervals, the grouped data will reveal the shape of the size distribution.

Table 1.1. Example of grouped data

Size range (μm)	Particle Count	Fraction/Size width (number/μm)	Particle Percent	Cumulative Percent
0.0-0.8	18	22.5	1.8	1.8
0.8-1.1	15	50	1.5	3.3
1.1-1.9	33	41.3	3.3	6.6
1.9-2.7	61	76.3	6.1	12.7
2.7-4.0	191	146.9	19.1	31.8
4.0-5.2	223	185.8	22.3	54.1
5.2-6.3	208	189.1	20.8	74.9
6.3-6.9	74	123.3	7.4	82.3
6.9-8.0	106	96.4	10.6	92.9
8.0-10	71	35.5	7.1	100
Total	1000		100.0	

One graphical representation of the grouped data is the histogram, shown in Figure 1.3, where the width of each rectangle represents the size interval and the height represents the number of particles in the interval.

Thus, doubling an interval's width results in roughly twice as many particles falling into that interval. To prevent this distortion, the histogram is normalized for interval width by dividing the number of particles in each interval by the width of that interval. The height of each rectangle now equals the number of particles per unit of size interval (number/μm) and the heights of intervals with different widths are comparable (Figure 1.4). Furthermore, the area of each rectangle is proportional to the number or frequency of particles in that size range.

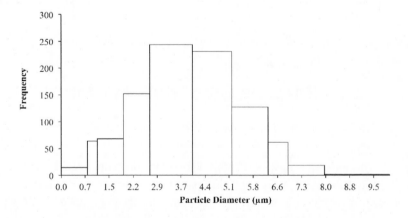

Figure 1.3. Histogram of frequency versus particle size.

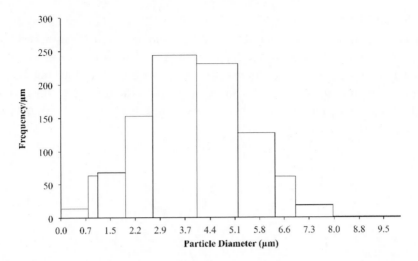

Figure 1.4. Frequency/μm versus particle size.

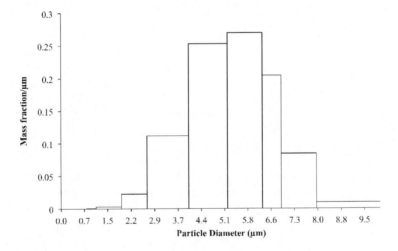

Figure 1.5 Mass distribution.

The height of the number divided by the size (y-axis) times with particle diameter (x-axis) gives an area equal to the number of particles in the interval. The area of all rectangles is the total number of particles.

The histogram is usually standardized for sample size by dividing the heights of the rectangles h_i (in frequency/μm) by the total number of particles observed in the sample, giving heights as fraction/μm. The area of each rectangle in the units of the graph, $h_i \Delta d_i$ is equal to the fraction f_i of particles in that size range, and the total area is equal to 1.0. This change allows for a direct comparison of histograms obtained from samples of different sizes.

As shown in Figure 1.4, the shape of the distribution is the same as that shown in Figure 1.3, but the ordinate is now the fraction of the total number of particles per unit of size interval. Since we describe the frequency function in terms of the particle size distribution, we can extend the analysis of size distribution by mass (Figure 1.5).

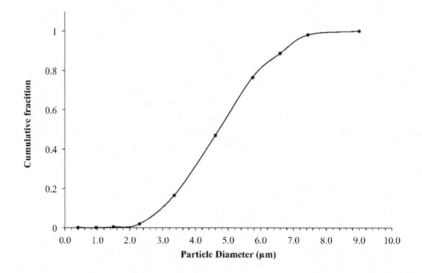

Figure 1.6. Cumulative mass distributions.

The cumulative distribution enables one to readily determine quantitative information about the particle size distribution (Figure 1.6). The fraction less than a given size can be read directly from the graph. The fraction of particles having diameters between two sizes can be determined directly by subtracting the cumulative fraction of one size from the other.

As a means for further summarizing the grouped data, a mathematical distribution function is assumed and parameters are calculated that define this function for a particular data set. Most distribution functions require two parameters: one that identifies the location or center of the distribution and one that characterizes the width or spread of the distribution. These parameters will be discussed elaborately in connection with specific distribution functions in subsequent sections.

The most commonly used quantities for defining the location of distribution are the mean, mode, and median. The mean or arithmetic average is simply the sum of all the particle sizes divided by the number of particles. The mean for the listed data is given by the midpoint size. The midpoint size can be a geometric mean or an arithmetic mean. The former is often preferred. The *median* is defined as the diameter that divides the frequency distribution curve into equal areas and the diameter corresponding to a cumulative fraction of 0.5.

The *mode* is the most frequent size on the frequency function curve. The mode can be determined by setting the derivative of the frequency function equal to zero and solving for *d*. For symmetrical distributions such as the normal distribution, the mean, median and mode will be the same value which is the diameter of the axis of symmetry. For an asymmetrical or skewed distribution, these quantities will have different values. The median is commonly used with skewed distributions because extreme values in the tail have less effect on the median than on the mean. Most aerosol size distributions are skewed, with a long tail to the right. For such a distribution, mode < median < mean.

The preceding sections have focused on the properties of the distributions of the size in general without considering any particular type of distribution. In this section, we describe the characteristics and applications of the log-normal distribution for aerosol particle size analysis (Figure 1.7). As discussed below, the normal distribution, although widely used elsewhere, is not suitable for most aerosol particle size distributions.

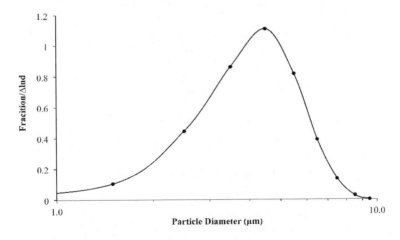

Figure 1.7. Frequency distribution curve (logarithmic size).

Other distributions have been applied to the aerosol particle sizes such as the Rosin-Rammler, power law, and exponential distributions. These distributions are applied to special situations but have limited application in aerosol science. The log-normal distributions have been selected empirically to fit the wide range and skewed shape of most aerosol size distributions. The normal distribution function is rarely used to describe aerosol particle size distributions because most aerosols exhibit a skewed distribution function (Figure 1.8). The normal distribution is, of course, symmetrical. It can be applied to monodisperse aerosols and to certain pollens and spores.

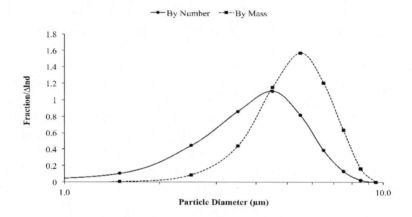

Figure 1.8. Count and mass distribution (logarithmic size).

The log-normal distribution is the most useful in situations where the distributed quantity can have only positive values and covers a wide range of values where the *ratio* of the largest to the smallest value is greater than 10. When this range is narrow, the log-normal distribution approximates the normal distribution.

The log-normal distribution is used extensively for aerosol size distributions because it fits the observed size distributions reasonably well and its mathematical form is convenient for dealing with the moment distributions and moment averages described in the preceding sections.

The standard deviation is replaced by the logarithms of the standard deviation, called the *geometric standard deviation* (GSD) or σ_g. The GSD is a dimensionless quality with a value equal to or greater than 1.0.

For the count distribution, the geometric mean diameter (d_g) is customarily replaced by the count median diameter (CMD). The geometric mean is the arithmetic mean of the distribution of $ln\ d_p$, which is a symmetrical normal distribution, and hence, its mean and median are equal. The median of the distribution of $ln\ d_p$ is also the median of the distribution of d_p, as the order of values does not change in converting to logarithms. Thus, for a log-normal count distribution, d_g = CMD. The frequency function can be expressed as a cumulative fraction.

Much of the practical application of the log-normal distribution to particle size analysis is facilitated by using log-probability graphs. In the most common form of these graphs, the axes are changed and the cumulative fraction (or percent) scale is converted to a probability scale (Figure 1.9). The probability scale compresses the percent scale near the median (50%) and expands the scale near the ends such that a cumulative plot of a log-normal distribution will yield a straight line. When the particle diameter scale is logarithmic, the graph is called a *log-probability plot.* When the size scale is linear, the cumulative graph will yield a straight line for a normal distribution and is called a *probability plot.* In either case, the median size can be read directly from the graph, as with any cumulative plot.

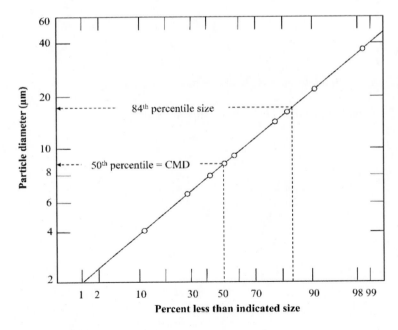

Figure 1.9. Log-probability graph.

A log-probability plot can be constructed on arithmetic graph paper by plotting the logarithm of the diameter versus the probits of the cumulative percentages. The latter, obtained from a table of probits, gives the linear displacement from the midpoint (50%) in units of standard deviations. The slope of the straight line is related to the GSD. A line with a steep slope is associated with a wide distribution and a line with a shallow slope represents a narrow distribution. A horizontal line in Figure 1.9 characterizes a monodisperse aerosol in which all particles have the same size.

For other expressions of a probability scale, it can be transformed with a Z-score (Figure 1.10). The particle size is transformed into a natural logarithm, and the frequency of data events is transformed to a Z-score, which is equal to the % cumulative of each data stage minus by the cumulative average and divided by the standard deviation of all interested events (Srichana, Suedee, and Srisudjai 2003). The slope of the linear equations is used to define the cut-off diameter ($Z=0$), d_{84} ($Z=1$), d_{16} ($Z=-1$) and GSDs are explained by the spread of the aerodynamic particle size distribution according to Equation 1.1.

$$GSD = \left(\frac{d_{84}}{d_{16}}\right)^{1/2}$$

(1.1)

where,

d_{84} is the diameter at 84% of the aerosol mass

d_{16} is the diameter at 16% of the aerosol mass

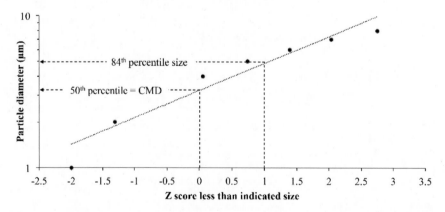

Figure 1.10. Log Z-score distribution.

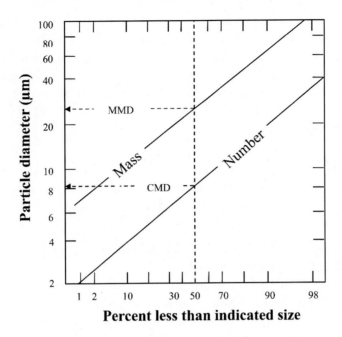

Figure 1.11. Cumulative number and cumulative mass distributions on the log-probability graph.

For any *normal* distribution, one standard deviation represents the *difference* between the size associated with a cumulative count of 84% and the median size (a cumulative count of 50%) or between the 50% cumulative size and the 16% cumulative size.

One great advantage of the log-normal distribution is that, for a given distribution, the GSD remains constant for all moment distributions.

Frequently in aerosol sampling, there is an aerodynamic size above which particles are aerodynamically unable to enter the sampling apparatus (Srichana, Martin, and Marriott 2000). This is called the *aerodynamic cut-off size*, which means that the cumulative line on the log-probability plot will curve near its upper end so that it never exceeds the cut-off size.

A similar limit may exist for the lower end of the size distribution if sizing is done by optical microscopy. Particles less than 0.3 μm in diameter are not included in the size distribution. This 0.3 μm limit, sometimes called the *optical cut-off*, curves the lower end of the size distribution line so that it never goes below 0.3 μm. These cut-offs are artifacts of the sampling and measurement system. If the cut-offs affect only a small fraction of the distribution, it is acceptable to ignore them when fitting a straight line to the data on a log-probability plot (Srichana, Suedee, and Srisudjai 2003).

Figure 1.11 shows both the number and mass distributions for the data given in Table 1.1, plotted as cumulative distributions on a log-probability graph paper. The horizontal axis refers to the cumulative percent of mass for the mass distribution line and the cumulative percent of the number distribution line.

1.4. The Hatch-Choate Conversion Equations

The real power of the log-normal distribution comes from the fact that any type of average diameter discussed in this chapter can easily be calculated for any known log-normal distribution that is a distribution for which one average diameter and the GSD are known. This is useful because it is frequently necessary to measure one characteristic of the size distribution, such as the number distribution, when what is really needed is another characteristic, such as the mass distribution or the diameter of the average mass.

$$d_g = size \, at \, 50\% cumulative \, frequency \tag{1.2}$$

$$\sigma_g = \frac{d_g}{size \, at \, 84\% oversize} \tag{1.3}$$

$$log \, d_{ln} = log \, d_g + 1.151 log^2 \sigma_g \tag{1.4}$$

$$log \, d'_g = log \, d_{ln} + 5.757 log^2 \sigma_g \tag{1.5}$$

Where,

d_g is a geometric mean diameter

σ_g is a geometric standard deviation

d_{ln} is a length-number mean diameter

d'_g is a geometric mean diameter on weight basis

If the distribution is log-normal, these quantities can be calculated directly using the log-normal conversion equations originally derived by Hatch and Choate (1929). These are known as the *Hatch-Choate equations.* The transformation equations were used to convert a number distribution to a weight distribution (Sinko 2006). The logarithm of the particle size can be plotted against the cumulative percent frequency on a log-probability scale (Equation 1.5).

Although these equations are written for number distributions, they can be combined to convert one type of average diameter to any other type of average diameter. The examples that follow are for the most common conversions between the number and mass distributions. Analogous equations can be written for any moment distribution, such as the distribution of surface area or of settling velocity.

1.5. Instrumentation in Particle Size Analysis

Drug particle size is recognized to play an important role in defining the location of the aerosol particle deposition in the respiratory tract (Hickey and Jones 2000). Therefore, a reliable technique is required in order to measure the particle size of the inhaled aerosols and to assess the drug deposition profiles both in terms of the quantity of the drug reaching the respiratory tract and its depth of penetration. When considering lung deposition, the aerodynamic diameter (D_{ae}) is of great interest. This is defined as the diameter of a unit density sphere with the same terminal settling velocity as the particle being studied (Hickey and Jones 2000, Mitchell and Nagel 2004).

Three main techniques are used to analyze the particle size of aerosols: direct imaging, optical sizing and inertial impaction (Hickey and Jones 2000).

1.5.1. Direct Imaging Based on Microscopy

The microscopic technique is a direct particle size measurement technique. The particle's morphology has been used to describe their powder properties via a number of approaches and mathematical models. Both qualitative and quantitative data have been determined by this technique to present simple to complex phenomena in DPIs. However, the subjective nature of the dimensions and the largely unrealistic and unrepresentative pattern of airway deposition are the limitations of this technique (Hickey and Jones 2000). A scanning electron microscope (SEM) is one type of microscope that produces images of a sample by scanning it with a focused beam of electrons. The electrons interact with atoms in the sample, producing various signals that contain information about the sample's surface topography and composition when it is equipped with an energy dispersive X-ray. The electron beam is generally scanned in a raster scan pattern, and the beam's position is combined with the detected signal to produce an image. SEM can achieve a resolution of better than 1 nanometer. Specimens can be observed in a high vacuum, low vacuum, wet conditions (in environmental SEM) and in a wide range of cryogenic or elevated temperatures. The most common SEM mode is the detection of secondary electrons emitted by atoms excited by the electron beam. The number of secondary electrons that can be detected depends on the angle at which the beam meets the surface of the specimen (i.e., on specimen topography). By scanning the sample and collecting the secondary electrons that are emitted using a special detector, an image displaying the topography of the surface is created. Here is an example of SEM micrographs obtained from a DPI formulation (Figure 1.12).

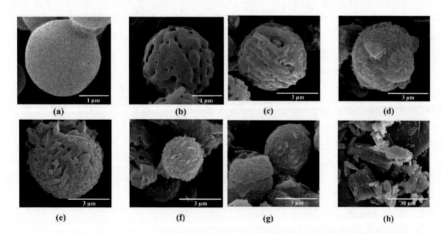

Figure 1.12. The scanning electron microscope (SEM) images of (a) spray dried mannitol (b) porous mannitol (c–g) Levofloxacin-proliposome formulations (h) Levofloxacin. (Reprinted from Rojanarat, W. et al., Pharmaceutics, 4(3), 385-412, 2012).

1.5.2 Optical Sizing

Light scattering (using laser particle sizing equipment) is a non-invasive technique which provides an estimate of volume median diameter and some index of polydispersity. The most notable of these methods used phase Doppler anemometry, time-of-flight laser velocimetry and laser diffraction. Each of these methods has an advantage of describing particles over a very broad range of sizes and therefore gives more information about the distributions in the absence of a chemical detection method. This is a drawback because the mass of a drug is related to its therapeutic effect. In addition, this technique does not take the anatomical structure of the human respiratory system into account (Hickey and Jones 2000).

When an electromagnetic beam is projected through a particle field, some portion of the beam is transmitted through the field while some portion of the beam is absorbed and the remaining is scattered by particles in the field. The ratio of the velocity of light in a vacuum to the velocity of light in a particular material is the refractive index of that material. For a given wavelength, the index of refraction depends only on the material, but it varies slightly with the wavelength of the light used.

In general, the distribution of light scattered by a particle is a function of the particle size and shape, the incident light and the reflection indices of both the particle and the surrounding medium (Kokhanovsky and Zege 1997). Both the scattering and absorption characteristics of a particle can be included by describing the particle's optical properties with a complex refractive index where the real part describes the scattered light characteristics and the imaginary part describes the absorption.

A laser beam is expanded and then collimated into a diameter of a few millimeters which passes through the particle cloud (Figure 1.13). Particles in the beam scatter in all directions, although predominantly in the near-forward direction. A receiving lens is used to focus both the transmitted beam and the forward scattered light (predominantly diffracted) onto a detector located at the back focal plane of the lens. The transmitted light is focused to a point on the optical axis, while the diffracted light forms a series of concentric rings.

As the receiving lens performs a Fourier transformation on the scattered light, light scattered at a given angle (θ) by a particle located anywhere in the illuminated sample volume will be focused at the same radial position in the transformed plane. Thus the resulting pattern is unaffected by the location of the particle or its motion.

Laser diffraction offers a convenient and established method to determine the particle size. It is used to determine a calibrant size either prior to or subsequent to entering through the impactor (Kwon et al. 2003, Ziegler and Wachtel 2005). Ziegler and Wachtel (2005) developed the laser diffraction method for particle size distribution measurements in pharmaceutical aerosols. An example of size measurement by laser diffraction is shown in Figure 1.14. It can be seen that the size distribution of the commercial powder is larger than the milled one. The milled powder has the median size around one micron whereas the commercial powder before milling has a median size of 4 microns with a range of 1-80 microns.

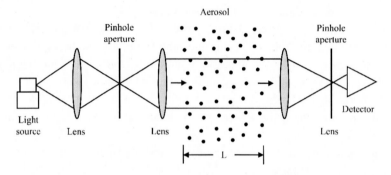

Figure 1.13. Schematic diagram of extinction-measuring apparatus.

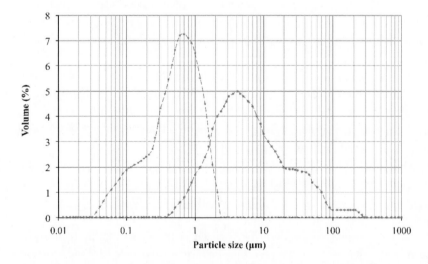

Figure 1.14. The particle size distribution obtained from laser diffraction of commercial powder (diamond red line) and milled powder (square blue line).

The parallel laser beam was introduced into a modified United States Pharmacopeia (USP) throat to measure particle distribution by a scattering pattern and intensity of light at different angles. The particle size distributions seem to be reproducible and have a strict correlation between the impactor and laser diffraction in the case of aqueous formulations (Ziegler and Wachtel 2005). Kwon et al. (2003) calibrated their 5-stage designed impactor using a gravimetric or counting method.

1.5.3. Inertial Sampling

This is the most widely used particle-size analysis method for inhaler output. Various instruments have been used to determine the particle size distribution of aerosols within a model respiratory tract designed to reproduce the anatomical dimension of an average healthy human airway. The instruments vary among inertial samplers, air inlet dimensions, the sampling airflow rates (12.5 to 120 LPM), the number of collecting stages (i.e. particle size ranges for collection within the distribution which varies from 2 to 8 stages) and the nature of the collection surface (liquid for impinger and uncoated or coated solid surfaces for the impactor). The drug is collected and washed from these stages and analyzed by chromatographic and spectrophotometric means to determine its mass (Hickey and Jones 2000).

A device with two stages has been developed as a quality control tool to indicate the proportion of the fine particles present in the distribution. The most frequently used *in vitro* method is a multiple-stage impactor because more information is recovered with regard to the range of particle sizes within the distribution. The cascade impactor utilizes the relationship between the velocity and the mass where larger particles with sufficient inertia are impacted on the upper stages whereas finer particles penetrate to the lower stages of the separator. Cascade impactors provide a useful aerodynamic measure of the distribution of particle sizes that can be used to compare devices and formulations. However, the disadvantage of this method is the narrow range of discriminated sizes, typically at values of D_{ae} from 0.2 to 10 μm, and requires considerable labor to perform the time-consuming analysis, which is subjected to operator variability and error (Hickey and Jones 2000).

To evaluate the deposition performance of a DPI *in vitro*, there are two common techniques, namely, a twin-stage impinger (TSI), which is official in the British Pharmacopeia (BP) (BP 2015), and an Andersen cascade impactor

(ACI), which has been approved by both the BP and the USP (Figure 1.15). The operation of the two techniques is described in Chapter 7.

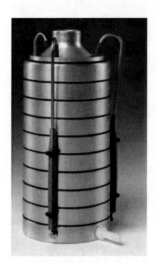 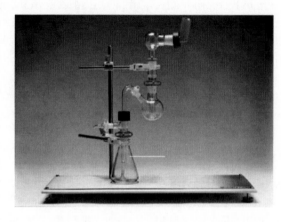

Figure 1.15. Andersen Cascade Impactor (left) and Twin Stage Impinger (right).

Twin Stage Impinger

The TSI is a two stage impinger that uses liquid at the first stage and a lower stage to capture the aerosol material while air with particles is drawn through the instrument. Even though the TSI method is easier to operate than the ACI method, limitations arise from the fact that the TSI divides the total spray into only two compartments. Hence, this method cannot discriminate between distributions with specific combinations of a size range and cannot precisely predict when operating out of the designed flow rate (Broadhead, Rouan, and Rhodes 1995, Geuns et al. 1997). The data derived from the TSI are intended to differentiate only good or bad formulations as determined by the fine particle fraction (FPF, particle size < 6.4 µm). This device is suitable for the quality control of aerosol products (Snell and Ganderton 1999). There was an attempt to integrate the oral throat cast to mimic the oropharynx while the USP describes a 90° sharp bend metal induction port to the cascade impactor system. Hence the rationale for the design of the *in vitro* test is an attempt to simulate the patient use as far as practicable with the hope of achieving a correlation of the results obtained from such tests with the *in vivo* performance (Srichana, Martin, and Marriott 1998).

Andersen Cascade Impactor

The ACI is a multistage and multi-orifice cascade impactor. The concept of the ACI evolved on the basis that the human respiratory tract represents an aerodynamic classifying system for airborne particulates. The ACI is comprised of eight aluminum stages which are held together by three spring clamps with o-ring seals. Each impactor stage contains multiple precision orifices so that when the air is drawn through the sampler, any airborne particles with high momentum were moved towards an impact with the collection plate for each stage and those with low momentum adjust to a new direction of flow and pass around the obstruction (Figure 1.16) (Hickey, Martonen, and Yang 1996).

DIRECTION OF AIRFLOW

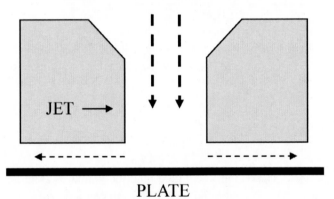

PLATE

Figure 1.16. General principle of inertial sampling through a jet onto a collection plate.

Table 1.2 presents the diameter of the orifices that are progressively smaller from the top to the bottom stages that range from 0.1004-inch diameter at stage 0 to 0.0100-inch diameter at stage 7. When operated at 28.3 LPM, the jet velocity is used to calculate the jet Reynolds number. The range of the particle sizes collected at each stage depends on the jet velocity of that stage and the cut-off diameter of the previous stage. Finally, the collected particles at each stage that are related to the aerodynamic dimension should be used to predict the deposition of the human lung airborne particles (USP 30-NF 25 2007).

**Table 1.2. Jet dimensions for each stage and
ACI (Mark II) parameters operating at 28.3 LPM.
(Adapted from Vaughan, NP., *Journal of Aerosol Science*, 1989)**

Stage	Orifice diameter (inches)	Number of orifices	Jet velocity (cm/s)	Re_j
0	0.1004	96	96.3	163.7
1	0.0743	96	175.8	221.2
2	0.0360	400	179.8	109.6
3	0.0280	400	297.2	140.9
4	0.0210	400	528.9	187.9
5	0.0135	400	1277.0	292.0
6	0.0100	400	2328.8	394.3
7	0.0100	201	4618.1	782.0
F	0.1100	Filter		

This simplified analysis is not accurate enough to characterize the impactor efficiency fully, but it does show that the Stokes number as defined by equation 1.6 is the relevant parameter for characterizing impaction.

$$Stk = \frac{\rho_p d_p^2 U_c}{9\eta D_j}$$
(1.6)

Every *in vitro* assessment technique must be validated. The performance of the inhaler device was reported as % FPF and Mass Median Aerodynamic Diameter (MMAD).

The characteristic dimension for the Stokes number of the impactor should be the distance between the jet and the impaction plate, but this is not the case. The streamlines at the nozzle exit are not strongly affected by the spacing between the nozzle and the plate because the jet of the aerosol expands only slightly until it reaches within about one jet diameter (D_j) of the impaction plate. Hence, the characteristic dimension for an impactor is the jet radius or half the width, rather than the spacing between the nozzle and the plate.

For most impactors, a complete curve of the collection efficiency versus particle size is not necessary. Impactors that have a "sharp cut-off" curve approach the ideal from the standpoint of particle size classification) step-function efficiency curve in which all particles greater than a certain aerodynamic size are collected and all particles less than that size pass through. The size in question is called the *cut-off size or cut-off diameter (d_{50})*.

As a practical matter, most well-designed impactors can be assumed to be ideal, and their efficiency curves are characterized by a Stokes number 50% (Stk_{50}) that provides a 50% collection efficiency. Stk_{50} is the location of the ideal cut-off curve that best fits the actual cut-off curve. This is equivalent to assuming that the mass of particles larger than the cut-off size that get through (the upper shaded area) equals the mass of particles below the cut-off size that are collected (the lower shaded area) (Figure 1.17).

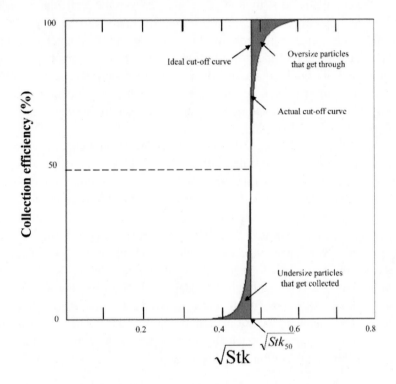

Figure 1.17. Actual and ideal impactor cut-off curves. (Adapted from Hinds, W. C., John Wiley & Sons, 2012).

All round jet impactors meeting these design criteria will have the same Stk_{50} value, regardless of the nozzle diameter. By adding a downstream filter to the impactor shown in Figure 1.18, one can collect all the particles that escape impaction. Sampling an aerosol with such an impactor can provide information about its particle size distribution. The mass of the particles collected on the impactor plate and of those collected on the filter are determined by weighing them before and after sampling. The impactor separates the sampled particulate mass into two particle size ranges that are contributed by particles larger than the cut-off size (collected on the impaction plate) and by particles smaller than the cut-off size (collected on the filter). For example, assume that an impactor with a 5 μm cut-off size collects 30% of the aerosol mass on the impactor plate and 70% on the filter. Then 30% of the aerosol mass is from particles greater than 5 μm in aerodynamic diameter and 70% is from particles less than 5 μm. Thus, this measurement provides one point on the cumulative distribution curve, that 70% of the particulate mass is associated with particles of less than 5 μm. By operating the impactor at several flow rates, each corresponding to a different cut-off diameter, several points on the cumulative mass distribution curve can be obtained. There are practical limitations on the range of flow rates that can be used and the aerosol size distribution must remain constant for all the samples. The latter problem can be overcome by simultaneously operating several impactors with different cut-off sizes.

The use of several impactors in parallel is, however not common because of the complexity of controlling multiple flow rates. The more common approach is to operate several impactors in series, arranged in order of decreasing cut-off size with the largest cut-off size first. This configuration is called a cascade impactor (Figure 1.18).

Each separate impactor is called an *impactor stage* (Figure 1.18). The cut-off size is reduced at each stage by decreasing the nozzle size. Reducing D_j increases U, and both serve to reduce d_{50} according to equation 1.7. Since the same volume of gas flows through each stage and only one flow needs to be controlled. Each stage is fitted with a removable impaction plate for gravimetric (or chemical) determination of the collected particles. The last stage in a cascade impactor is usually followed by a filter that captures all particles less than the cut-off size of that stage.

$$d_{50} = \frac{9\eta D_j Stk_{50}}{\rho_p U} \qquad (1.7)$$

In its operation, each stage is assumed to capture all particles reaching it that are larger than its cut-off size. Because the aerosol flows in sequence through successive stages, the particles captured on the impaction plate of a given stage represent all particles smaller than the cut-off size of the previous stage and larger than the cut-off size of the given stage. It is important to keep in mind that an impactor stage consists of a nozzle section and the impaction plate (Figure 1.16).

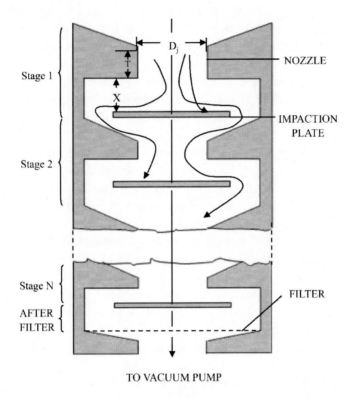

Figure 1.18. Schematic diagram of cascade impactor with nozzle and impaction plate.

Data reduction is based on the assumption that each stage has the ideal cut-off characteristics. This assumption imposes an additional requirement that the cut-off sizes for successive stages be far enough apart that there is a negligible overlap in their collection curves. If they overlap, a much more complicated analysis is required, using the exact shape of the collection efficiency curve. Also, it is assumed that the non-ideal cut-off effects cancel out; that is, the mass of the oversized particles getting through each stage equals the mass of undersized ones that are collected. This may not always be the case and if it is not this will cause a distortion of the size distribution.

The cut-off size ranges given are for typical flow rates and can be changed by operating the impactor at a different flow rate according to equation 1.7. The preceding discussion has assumed that the particles stick if they strike the surface of the impaction plate. For liquid particles, this is nearly always correct. Solid particles, however, may bounce and blow off when they strike the impaction plate, or they may adhere. Some of the mass of a certain particle size ends up on a lower stage and is thus attributed to a smaller particle size range. Furthermore, once a particle bounces it is likely to continue to bounce in subsequent stages because the impaction velocity is greater in these stages. Whether or not a particle bounces depends on its material, its velocity and the type of impaction surface. Coating the impaction plate with a thin film of oil or grease reduces bounce (Hinds 2012). Antibounce coatings have been used successfully including high-vacuum grease, petroleum jelly, and silicone oil. To obtain a thin film, these materials are usually dissolved in solvents such as toluene or cyclohexane and are painted or sprayed onto the impaction surface, and allowed to dry. Even with an antibounce coating, bounce can occur when the impaction surface becomes overloaded with particles. This is because incoming particles have an increased probability of impacting on a deposited particle rather than the coating. Impaction surfaces made up of a porous metal, or a coarse filter saturated with oil served as a reservoir and allowed the oil to "wick" through the deposited particles to maintain an effective antibounce coating. Plastic films or small pore membrane filters do not reduce particle rebound, although these surfaces may be convenient for analytical purposes.

Particles can be deposited in the passageways between stages of the cascade impactor. Such deposition is called the interstage loss and represents another operational problem with cascade impactors. For conventional cascade impactors, interstage losses are primarily a problem of large particles being lost in the first two stages. Particles are lost primarily by inertial removal at bends in the flow path. Since these interstage losses depend on particle size and are not included in the collected mass, they distort the size distribution toward smaller sizes. Interstage losses can be reduced by designing the impactor to minimize sharp bends in the interstage flow path of the first few stages or by operating the impactor at a lower flow rate. As particles deposit on the impaction plate, they form a spot that grows into a conical pile of powder that changes the flow geometry and the cut-off size. This also reduces the effectiveness of any grease coatings and sets a practical upper limit on the mass that can be collected on any stage. The lower limit is usually set by the analytical technique used, such as the sensitivity of the balance used. Some impactors are equipped with a preseparator to collect large amounts of the large particles so that accurate measurements can be made of the size distribution in the smaller particle size range. Preseparators do not need to have a sharp cut-off, because as long as the preseparator collects particles larger than the cut-off size at the first stage, the mass collected by the preseparator can be combined with that collected on the first stage to give the total mass that was larger than the first-stage cut-off size. Some impactors have a collection surface that slowly rotates during operation, to prevent excessive buildup of deposited particles. Dechraksa et al., (2014) developed a validated computational fluid dynamic (CFD) model of the ACI and investigated the effects of the preseparator on the CFD parameters. The flow field indicated that the preseparator accelerated the airflow velocity at the induction tube. The CFD model explained the airflow of the preseparator equipped model by accelerating the airflow along the inlet port to maximize the trapping of the desirable particles and the generation of a smooth wall shear stress at the collection plate to reduce the particle reentrainment. Figure 1.19 shows a particle size distribution of isoniazid DPIs evaluated by the ACI at a flow rate of 60 LPM. The drug particles deposited mainly on the glass throat (GT) and the preseparator. The drug particles traveled deeper into the impactor stage -1 to stage 6. It was predicted that the smaller drug particles were likely to reach the lower airways.

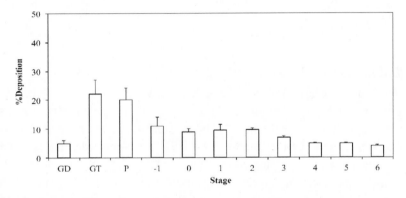

Figure 1.19. The particle size distribution of an isoniazid dry powder inhaler after aerosolization into the ACI at the flow rate of 60 LPM (GD = Glass Device, GT = Glass Throat, P = Preseparator) (mean ± SD, n = 3).

Next Generation Impactor (NGI)

The next generation impactor (Figure 1.20) or Apparatus 5 for DPIs in the USP (USP 30-NF 25 2007) was first designed in 2000 to evaluate pharmaceutical aerosols. This is highly accurate and easy to operate. There is a linear correlation between the data obtained from the ACI and NGI (Guo et al. 2008) at 30 LPM. Variations due to manual actuation (operator variance), flow rates and induction ports, significantly affect the particle size distribution (PSD) and dose delivery profile. The instrument can be operated at a flow rate of 15-100 LPM. There are 7 stages (cut-off diameters are 0.54-6.12 μm). The unit easily collects samples, and the interstage loss is low. Each stage has 500 < Re < 3000.

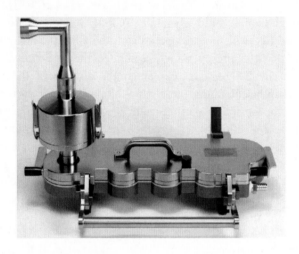

Figure 1.20. Next generation impactor.

Multistage Liquid Impinger (MSLI)

This impinger has combined the ACI and TSI and reduced the number of stages to only 4-5 stages (Figure 1.21). It is operated by the concept of aerosol particles being trapped by the liquid. The instrument can be operated at 30-100 LPM as stated in the USP apparatus 4 for DPI. It can be used either with DPI, MDI or nebulizer. BP recommended that the MSLI be operated at 60 LPM. The cut-off diameters of stages 1, 2, 3 and 4 were 13, 6.8, 3.1 and 1.7 μm, respectively. Stage 5 collects particles with sizes less than 1.7 μm. This technique reduces the re-entrainment of aerosol particles.

Figure 1.22 shows the particle distribution of two DPI formulations of budesonide after aerosolization into the MSLI at 60 LPM into two different inspiratory volumes of 1 and 2 L. The mass deposition on each stage of the MSLI was not different between the two different inspiratory volumes. Hence, the inspiratory volume at the first few seconds is crucial.

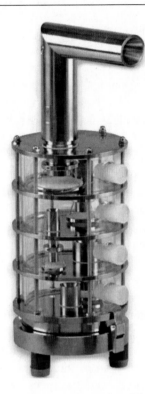

Figure 1.21. Multistage liquid impinger from Copley Scientific.

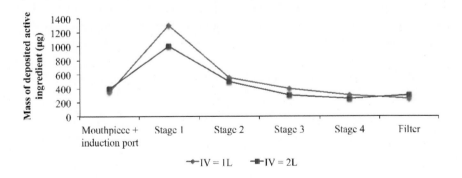

Figure 1.22. Aerodynamic particle size distributions of budesonide in the test formulation with inspiratory volumes (IV) of 1 and 2 L.

1.5.4. Time-of-Flight Instruments

Time-of-flight instruments can provide real-time, high-resolution measurements of aerodynamic particle size and size distribution over a wide size range. Air is accelerated (> 10^6 m/s^2) in a converging nozzle to a high velocity (> 100 m/s) at the nozzle exit. Two narrowly focused laser beams are positioned in the jet about 100 μm apart (Figure 1.23). Particles, focused into the center of the jet by the clean sheath air, are accelerated by the airflow in the nozzle. Small particles less than 0.3 μm can keep up with the accelerating air in the nozzle and exit with approximately the same velocity as the air. As a particle passes through the first laser beam, it creates a very brief (1μs) pulse of scattered light that is detected by a photomultiplier tube. A similar pulse is generated when the particle passes through the second beam. The time interval between the two pulses is sensed electronically and is used to determine the average velocity of the particle as it passes through the space between the two laser beams. The time between these two beams is measured with a precision of 25 nanoseconds and is termed the time of flight (TOF). Since TOF is dependent on particle size, it is possible to obtain a particle size distribution of any powder including, for example, the lactose and drug depositing on the individual plates of an ACI after a dry powder formulation has been aerosolized into the impactor. With suitable calibration, the particle's aerodynamic diameter can be determined from the magnitude of the TOF. This is done electronically and the particle size and size distribution are determined nearly in real time. There are important limitations to these instruments that arise primarily because particle motion is outside the Stokes region due to the high velocities used.

The general form of the force equation is given by equation 1.8.

$$C_d \frac{\pi d^2}{4} \rho_a \frac{\left(V_a - V_p\right)^2}{2} = \frac{1}{6} \pi d^3 \rho_p \frac{dv}{dt} \tag{1.8}$$

where:

C_d = drag coefficient d = particle diameter (cm)

ρ_a = density of air (g mL^{-1}) ρ_p = density of particle (g mL^{-1})

V_a = air velocity (dyne s cm^3) V_p = particle velocity (cm s^{-1})

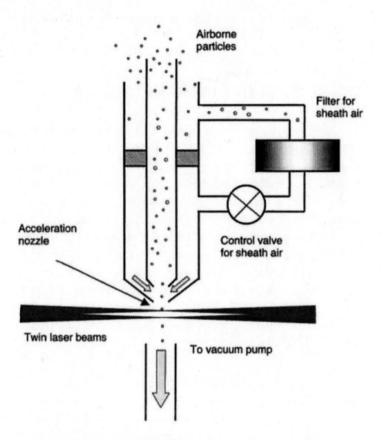

Figure 1.23. Time of flight mass spectrometry size analysis. (Adapted from https://www.osapublishing.org).

The term $C_d \dfrac{\pi d^2}{4}$ relates to the drag coefficient and projected area of the

particle, while the term $\rho_a \dfrac{\left(V_a - V_p\right)^2}{2}$ relates to the air density and

differential velocity of the air and the particle. The right side of the equation is simply the particle volume multiplied by the density $\left(\dfrac{1}{6}\pi d^3 \rho_p\right)$ and yields

the particle mass, which is then multiplied by the particle acceleration $\left(\dfrac{dv}{dt}\right)$.

1.6. Isokinetic Sampling

Isokinetic sampling is a procedure to ensure that a representative sample of aerosol enters the inlet of a sampling tube when sampling from a moving aerosol stream. The sampling may be extracted from a windy environment by a probe. Sampling is isokinetic when the inlet axis of the sampler, a thin-walled tube or probe, is aligned parallel to the gas streamlines and the gas velocity entering the probe equals the free-stream velocity approaching the inlet. This condition is equivalent to taking a sample so that there is no distortion of the streamlines just upstream of the inlet (Figure 1.24). If sampling is isokinetic, there is no particle loss at the inlet, regardless of the particle size or inertia. Isokinetic sampling in no way ensures that there are no losses between the inlet and the collector; instead, it guarantees that the concentration and size distribution of the aerosol entering the tube are the same as that in the flowing stream.

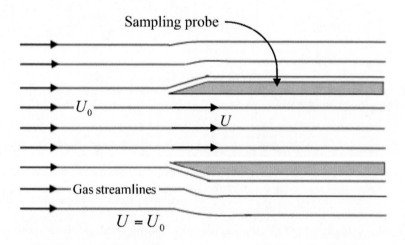

Figure 1.24. Isokinetic sampling.

In isokinetic sampling, failure to sample isokinetically may result in a distortion of the size distribution and a biased estimate of the concentration. These effects arise because of particle inertia in the region of curved streamlines near the inlet. Depending on the conditions, the sample may contain an excess or a deficiency of large particles. If sampling is not done isokinetically, there is no way to determine the true concentration unless the original particle size distribution is known or can be estimated.

1.7. The *In Vivo* Assessment Technique

The *in vivo* assessment technique is commonly used in human volunteers. There are 2 common techniques including a pharmacokinetic-pharmacodynamic measurement and gamma scintigraphy.

Pharmacokinetic data (plasma and urine levels) and pharmacodynamic data (e.g., pharmacological response heart rate or blood pressure) are sometimes used to infer the delivery of asthma medications to the lungs (Kempsford et al. 2005). However, only classical bioequivalence testing based upon equal rates and extents of drug absorption is inappropriate to show the equivalence of products containing inhaled asthma drugs that act directly on the airway surface. Further, this technique needs to be validated and is probably applicable only in a limited range of pharmaceuticals.

Another *in vivo* assessment method is the non-invasive imaging technique such as gamma scintigraphy. A method of wide application to radiolabelling dry powders is by adsorbing the radiolabel on the active particles in a suitable liquid. This is achieved by wetting the drug particles with a nonsolvent containing the radiolabel, followed by the evaporation of the solvent, leaving the radiolabel on the surface of the drug particles. This method gives a measure of local bioavailability at the site of action in the lungs and the lung deposition data are strongly correlated with the clinical response to the inhaled asthma drugs (Newman and Wilding 1998). However, all of the *in vivo* assessment techniques are not easy to monitor in product development processes; therefore, *in vitro* assessments are still necessary.

References

BP. 2015. *British Pharmacopoeia*. London: Pharmaceutical Press.

Broadhead, Joanne, Edmond S. K. Rouan, and Christopher T. Rhodes. 1995. "Dry-powder inhalers: evaluation of testing methodology and effect of inhaler design." *Pharmaceutica Acta Helvetiae* 70 (2):125-31.

Dechraksa, Janwit, Tan Suwandecha, Kittinan Maliwan, and Teerapol Srichana. 2014. "The comparison of fluid dynamics parameters in an Andersen cascade impactor equipped with and without a preseparator." *AAPS PharmSciTech* 15 (3):792-801. doi: 10.1208/s12249-014-0102-2.

Geuns, Eduard R. M., Johan S. Toren, Dirk M. Barends, and Auke Bult. 1997. "Decrease of the stage-2 deposition in the twin impinger during storage of beclomethasone dipropionate dry powder inhalers in controlled and uncontrolled humidities." *European Journal of Pharmaceutics and Biopharmaceutics* 44 (2):187-194. doi: 10.1016/S0939-6411(97)00072-6.

Guo, Changning, Stacey R Gillespie, John Kauffman, and William H Doub. 2008. "Comparison of delivery characteristics from a combination metered-dose inhaler using the Andersen cascade impactor and the next generation pharmaceutical impactor." *Journal of Pharmaceutical Sciences* 97 (8):3321-3334.

Hatch, Theodore, and Sarah P. Choate. 1929. "Statistical description of the size properties of non uniform particulate substances." *Journal of the Franklin Institute* 207 (3):369-387. doi: 10.1016/S0016-0032(29)91451-4.

Hickey, Anthony J. 2004. *Pharmaceutical Inhalation Aerosol Technology*. 2nd ed. Broken Sound Parkway NW: CRC Press.

Hickey, Anthony J., and Latarsha D. Jones. 2000. "Particle-size analysis of pharmaceutical aerosols." *Pharmaceutical Technology* 24 (9):48-50.

Hickey, Anthony J., Ted B. Martonen, and Yadong Yang. 1996. "Theoretical relationship of lung deposition to the fine particle fraction of inhalation aerosols." *Pharm Acta Helv* 71 (3):185-90.

Hinds, William C. 2012. *Aerosol Technology: Properties, Behavior, and Measurement of Airborne Particles*: John Wiley & Sons.

Kempsford, Rodger, Malcom Handel, Rashmi Mehta, Mariza De Silva, and Peter Daley-Yates. 2005. "Comparison of the systemic pharmacodynamic effects and pharmacokinetics of salmeterol delivered by CFC propellant and non-CFC propellant metered dose inhalers in healthy subjects." *Respiratory Medicine CME* 99 Suppl A:S11-9. doi: 10.1016/j.rmed.2004.11.005.

Kokhanovsky, Alexander A., and Eleonora P. Zege. 1997. "Optical properties of aerosol particles: A review of approximate analytical solutions." *Journal of Aerosol Science* 28 (1):1-21. doi: 10.1016/S0021-8502(96)00058-4.

Kwon, Su B., Keong S. Lim, Ji S. Jung, Gwi N. Bae, and Ki W. Lee. 2003. "Design and calibration of a 5-stage cascade impactor (K-JIST cascade impactor)." *Journal of Aerosol Science* 34 (3):289-300. doi: 10.1016/S0021-8502(02)00177-5.

Mitchell, Jolyon, and Mark Nagel. 2004. "Particle size analysis of aerosols from medicinal inhalers." *KONA Powder and Particle Journal* 22 (3):32-65. doi: 10.14356/kona.2004010.

Newman, Stephen P, and Ian R. Wilding. 1998. "Gamma scintigraphy: an in vivo technique for assessing the equivalence of inhaled products." *International Journal of Pharmaceutics* 170 (1):1-9. doi: 10.1016/S0378-5173(98)00029-5.

Rojanarat, Wipaporn, Titpawan Nakpheng, Ekawat Thawithong, Niracha Yanyium, and Teerapol Srichana. 2012. "Levofloxacin-proliposomes: opportunities for use in lung tuberculosis." *Pharmaceutics* 4 (3):385-412.

Sinko, Patrick. 2006. *Martin's Physical Pharmacy and Pharmaceutical Sciences: Physical Chemical and Biopharmaceutical Principles in the Pharmaceutical Sciences.* Edited by PJ. Sinko. 6th ed. Baltimore, MD: Lippincott Williams & Wilkin.

Snell, Noel, and David Ganderton. 1999. "Assessing lung deposition of inhaled medications." *Respiratory Medicine CME* 93 (2):123-33.

Srichana, Teerapol, Gary P. Martin, and Christopher M. Marriott. 2000. "A human oral-throat cast integrated with a twin-stage impinger for evaluation of dry powder inhalers." *Journal of Pharmacy and Pharmacology* 52 (7):771-778.

Srichana, Teerapol, Gary P. Martin, and Christopher Marriott. 1998. "Calibration method for the Andersen cascade impactor." *Journal of Aerosol Science* 29 (SUPPL.2):S761-S762.

Srichana, Teerapol, Roongnapa Suedee, and P. Srisudjai. 2003. "Application of spectrofluorometry for evaluation of dry powder inhalers *in vitro*." *Pharmazie* 58 (2):125-9.

USP 30-NF 25. 2007. *United States Pharmacopeia and National Formulary (USP 30-NF 25).* 39 ed. Vol. 2. Rockville, MD: United States Pharmacopeia Convention.

Vaughan, Nicholas. 1989. "The Andersen impactor: calibration, wall losses and numerical simulation." *Journal of Aerosol Science* 20 (1):67-90.

Ziegler, Jochen, and Herbert Wachtel. 2005. "Comparison of cascade impaction and laser diffraction for particle size distribution measurements." *Journal of Aerosol Medicine* 18 (3):311-24. doi: 10.1089/jam.2005.18.311.

Chapter 2

Flow Properties

2.1. Introduction

In many situations in aerosol technology, there is an interaction between the particles and the gas, and one must take into account the discontinuous nature of the gas. That is, the gas cannot be treated as a continuous fluid but must be considered as an ensemble of rapidly moving molecules colliding randomly with the particles.

The criterion for using such an approach depends on the particle size relative to the spacing between the gas molecules. Instead of the average spacing between molecules, a more useful concept is the *mean free path*, which is defined as the average distance traveled by a molecule between successive collisions. The mean free path of a gas can be determined from the average number of collisions a particular molecule undergoes in one second and the average distance it has traveled in that second.

2.2. Reynolds Number

A key to understanding the aerodynamic properties of aerosol particles is the Reynolds number (R_e) which is a dimensionless number that characterizes the fluid flow through a pipe or around an obstacle such as an aerosol particle.

The Reynolds number has the following properties:

1. It is an index of the flow regime to provide a benchmark that will determine whether the fluid flow is laminar or turbulent.
2. It is proportional to the ratio of the inertial forces to the viscous forces acting on each element of the fluid. This ratio is the key to determine which flow resistance equation is correct in a given situation.
3. Equality of the Reynolds numbers is required for a geometrically similar flow to occur around geometrically similar objects. This similarity means that the pattern of the streamlines will be the same for flow around different-sized objects or even the flow of different fluids. A streamline is the path traced by a tiny element of fluid as it flows around an obstacle.

The Reynolds number can be derived by the ratio of the inertial force to a viscous force acting on an element of fluid in a steady-flow system. The *viscous force* is defined by the air viscosity.

$$R_e = \frac{\rho V d}{\eta} \tag{2.1}$$

Table 2.1. Property of air at standard conditions:
293K, 101kPa (20°C, 760 mmHg)

Property	SI Units	cgs Units
Viscosity	1.81×10^{-4} Pa·s (N·s/m²)	1.81×10^{-4} dyne·s/cm²
Density	1.20 Kg/m³	1.20×10^{-3} g/cm³
Diffusion Coefficient	2×10^{-5} m²/s	0.20 cm²/s
Mean Free Path	0.066 µm	0.066 µm

The Reynolds number is dimensionless in any consistent system of units. The quantities associated with inertia are in the numerator and viscosity is in the denominator. It is important to note that the density is that of the gas and not the aerosol particles.

The properties of air given in Table 2.1 provide a simpler form of the Reynolds number for use with SI or cgs units at standard conditions.

Equation 2.1 applies equally well to flow in a pipe or particle motion; the latter is called the *particle Reynolds number.*

The Reynolds number depends only on the relative velocity between an object such as an aerosol particle and surrounding gas. It is aerodynamically equivalent for the air to flow past a stationary particle or for the particle to move through the stationary air at the same velocity. *Laminar flow* around a particle occurs at low Reynolds numbers (Re < 1), for which the viscous forces are much greater than the inertial forces. This kind of flow is characterized by a smooth pattern of streamlines that are symmetrical on the upstream and downstream sides of the particle (Figure 2.1(a)). As a Reynolds number increases above 1.0, eddies are formed downstream.

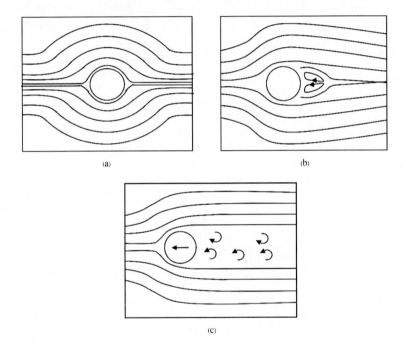

(a)

(b)

(c)

Figure 2.1. Flow around a sphere. (a) Laminar flow R_e = 0.1. (b) Turbulent flow R_e = 2. (c) Turbulent flow R_e = 250.

The Reynolds number is also important in an *in vitro* experiment of aerosol deposition. The complexity of extrathoracic airways leads to different Reynolds numbers that affect the aerosol deposition pattern (Ma and Darquenne 2011). Therefore, a correction in the Reynolds number is a critical step to develop an *in vitro* model for aerosol assessment (Nicolaou and Zaki 2013).

A *flow controller* combines a pressure regulator with a metering valve to maintain a constant flow rate under varying conditions. The regulator maintains a constant pressure drop across the metering valve.

Unlike the variable-head meter that measures a pressure drop varying with flow rate, the variable orifice area with the flow rate will maintain a nearly constant pressure drop. The most common type of variable area meter is the *rotameter* (Figure 2.2) that consists of a float that is free to move up and down in a vertical, tapered tube through which the fluid to be measured passes.

The float rises in the tapered tube until its weight balances the upward drag force due to the fluid flowing up through the tube. The area between the float and the tube wall increases as the float rises, and reduces the velocity and drag force of the fluid.

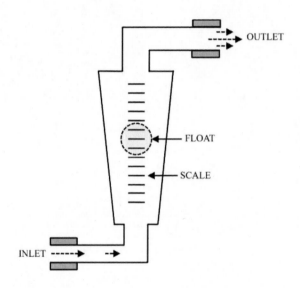

Figure 2.2. Rotameter.

2.3. Uniform Particle Motion

The most common and perhaps the most important type of particle motion is steady, straight-line motion. This uniform motion is typically the result of the action of two forces, a constant external force such as gravity or an electrical force and the resistance of the gas to particle motion. Analysis of a uniform particle motion is especially useful for the study of aerosols because in most situations aerosol particles come to a constant velocity almost instantly. The resisting force of the gas depends on the relative velocity between the particle and the gas and is the same whether the particle moves through the gas or the gas flows past the particle.

The general equation for the force that resists the motion of a sphere passing through a gas was derived by Newton as part of a ballistic evaluation of cannon balls.

Newton's resistance equation is valid for a wide range of particle motion but is useful primarily for Reynolds numbers that are greater than 1,000 but not to aerosol particles. As discussed earlier, Stokes' law, although derived from first principles, represents a special case of Newton's resistance law.

Newton indicated that the resistance encountered by a cannon ball passing through the air is a result of the breakup of the air that has to be pushed aside to allow the sphere to travel through it. In one second, a sphere of diameter d will push aside a volume of gas equal to the projected area of the sphere multiplied by its velocity (V).

The mass $(\dot{m})$ of this amount of gas is,

$$\dot{m} = \rho_g \frac{\pi}{4} d^2 V \tag{2.2}$$

Acceleration of the displaced gas is proportional to a relative velocity between the sphere and the gas, and thus the change of momentum per unit time is,

$$\frac{change\ of\ momentum}{unit\ time} \alpha\, \dot{m}V = \rho_g \frac{\pi}{4} d^2 V^2 \tag{2.3}$$

By definition, this rate of change of momentum is equal to the force required to move the sphere through the gas, the *gas resistance* or *drag force* is given by

$$F_D = K \rho_g \frac{\pi}{4} d^2 V^2 \tag{2.4}$$

Where K is a constant of proportionality. Newton originally thought that K was independent of the velocity for a given shape. This is true, however, only when the Reynolds number for particle motion is greater than 1,000. This is the general form of the resistance equation that is valid for all subsonic motions of particles. The dimensionless coefficient of drag is constant for spheres having $R_e > 1,000$.

The derivation of equation 2.4 is based on the inertia of the gas, and it follows that equation 2.3 is valid only for motion at high Reynolds numbers, where the inertial forces are much larger than the viscous forces.

Since most aerosol motion problems have either a diameter or a velocity as one of the unknowns, the Reynolds number cannot be calculated until the problem is solved.

$$F_D = C_D \frac{\pi}{8} \rho_g d^2 V^2 \tag{2.5}$$

$$C_D = \frac{24}{R_e}(1 + 0.15 \cdot R_e^{0.687}) \tag{2.6}$$

Newton's drag ($R_e > 1,000$) applies to a particle motion for which the viscous effects of the gas can be neglected compared with the inertial effects. In 1851, Stokes derived an expression for drag at the other extreme when inertial forces are negligible compared to viscous forces. As mentioned, the Reynolds number is a ratio of inertial to viscous forces; consequently, a condition of negligible inertial forces compared to viscous forces implies a low Reynolds number and laminar flow. Because of the low velocities and small particle sizes involved, most aerosol motion occurs at low Reynolds numbers. Stokes' law thus has wide application for the study of aerosols, and it is worthwhile reviewing the derivation of the law and its assumptions and implications.

Stokes' law is a solution for the generally unsolvable Navier-Stokes equations. These equations are the general differential equations that describe fluid motion. They are derived from the application of Newton's second law to a fluid element on which the gravity, pressure, and viscous forces are acting. The resulting equations are very difficult to solve because they are nonlinear, partial differential equations.

In general, some simplifying assumptions must be made before they can be solved. Stokes solution does this by assuming that the inertial forces are negligible compared to the viscous forces. This assumption eliminates the higher order terms in the Navier-Stokes equations and yields linear equations that can be solved. Further assumptions of Stokes derivation are incompressible fluid, no walls or other particles nearby, constant motion of the particle, rigid spheres and zero fluid velocity at the particle's surface.

Stokes solved the Navier-Stokes equations with the assumptions just stated to obtain equations for the forces acting at any point in the fluid surrounding a spherical particle. The net force acting on the particle was obtained by integrating the normal and tangential forces over the surface of the particle. The two resulting forces acting in the direction opposite to the particle motion are the *form component,*

$$F_n = \pi \eta V d \tag{2.7}$$

and the *frictional component.*

$$F_\tau = 2\pi \eta V d \tag{2.8}$$

These components are combined to give the total resisting force on a spherical particle moving with a velocity V through a fluid. This is *Stokes' law.* When the resisting force is experienced by a particle, it can be described by equation 2.9 and the motion of the particles is said to be in the Stokes region.

$$F_D = 3\pi \eta V d \tag{2.9}$$

As a particle moves through a fluid, it deforms the fluid, causing layers of the fluid in the region around the particle to slide over one another. The resisting force is the result of the friction of these layers sliding over one another. The energy spent overcoming this resistance is dissipated as heat throughout the fluid. In practice, the use of Stokes' law is restricted to situations in which the particle Reynolds number is less than 1.0. At a Reynolds number of 1.0, the error in the drag force calculated by Stokes' law is 12% and at a Reynolds number of 0.3 it is 5%.

It is instructive to compare the drag force given by Stokes' law with that given by Newton's law. Stokes' law contains viscosity, but not factors associated with inertia. Newton's law contains ρ_g but not viscosity. Solving equation 2.9 for the coefficient of drag gives

$$F_D = 3\pi\eta Vd = C_D \frac{\pi}{8} \rho_g d^2 V^2 \text{, for } R_e < 1 \tag{2.10}$$

This is the equation for the straight-line portion at the left of Figure 2.1. Because equation 2.10 includes V and d, it changes the functional relationship of Newton's equation from an equation having a drag force proportional to V^2 and d^2 to one with a drag force that is proportional to V and d according to Stokes' law (Theerachaisupakij et al. 2002). For conditions between the range of application of Newton's and Stokes' laws, the functional dependence of drag gradually changes from V^2 to V and from d^2 to d. This is the curved portion of Figure 2.1. The frictional component, equation 2.8, represents two-thirds of the Stokes drag, and the expression is equivalent to equation 2.10 for the flow in tubes where there is no form component and gives $C_0 = \dfrac{16}{R_e}$, or two-thirds of equation 2.10.

How do the other assumptions of Stokes' law limit its application to aerosol particles? The assumption of an incompressible fluid implies that air is compressible, but rather that it does not compress significantly near the particle as the particle moves through it. This is equivalent to assuming that the relative velocity is much less than the speed of sound, which is nearly always the case for aerosol particles.

The presence of a wall within 10 diameters of a particle will modify the drag force on the particle. Because of the small size of the aerosol particles, only a tiny fraction of the aerosol particles will be within 10 particle diameters of a wall in any real container or tube.

The correction to Stokes' law for non-rigid spheres such as water droplets is generally insignificant. Water droplets settle 0.6% faster than predicted by the Stokes' law because of circulations that develop within the droplet caused by the resisting force at the droplet surface.

$$C_D = \frac{24\eta}{\rho_g Vd} = \frac{24}{R_e} \tag{2.11}$$

In addition to Stokes' law which is a simplified version of the Navier-Stokes equations, the advancement in computational power enabled a full numerical solving of the Navier-Stokes equations using a simulation of the computational fluid dynamics (CFD). The CFD can deal with the laminar flow or turbulence flow problems by coupling with a turbulence model such as k-ε and k-ω models. A sophisticated full-scale CFD simulation of the Andersen cascade impactor (ACI) can visualize flow field and the aerodynamic parameters that affect the motion of the particles inside the impactor (Figure 2.3) (Dechraksa et al. 2014). The streamline velocity at stage 0 showed a different clustering pattern for the high velocity where the streamline velocity was in the traditional induction port (Figure 2.3a, b) and exhibited a higher airflow velocity than that in the preseparator (Figure 2.3c, d) for both flow rates (28.3 and 60 LPM).

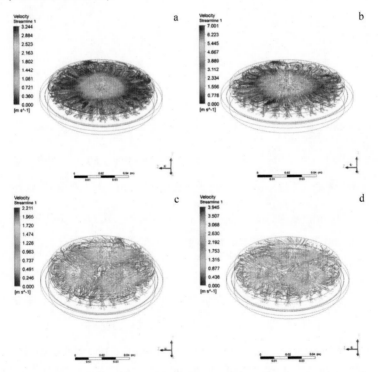

Figure 2.3. Airflow visualization in the ACI at stage 0 under different inlet profiles. (a) Stage 0 under a traditional induction port at 28.3 LPM. (b) Stage 0 under a traditional induction port at 60 LPM. (c) Stage 0 under a preseparator at 28.3 LPM. (d) Stage 0 under preseparator at 60 LPM. (Reprinted from Dechraksa, J. et al., AAPS PharmSciTech, 15(3), 792-801, 2014. With the permission from Springer).

2.4. Settling Velocity and Mechanical Mobility

One important application of Stokes' law is the determination of the velocity of an aerosol particle undergoing gravitational settling in still air. When a particle is traveling in air, it reaches the terminal settling velocity very quickly. Under constant velocity conditions, the drag force on the particle is equal and opposite to the force of gravity F_G.

$$F_D = F_G = mg \tag{2.12}$$

$$3\pi\eta V d = \frac{(\rho_P - \rho_g)\pi d^3 g}{6} \tag{2.13}$$

Where, g is the acceleration of gravity, ρ_P is the density of the particle and ρ_g is the density of the gas. The latter has been included to account for the buoyancy effect, but this can be neglected because ρ_P is much greater than ρ_g. For example, a water droplet settling in the air has a density ratio $\rho / \rho_g = 800$ and neglecting buoyancy introduces an error of only 0.1%. Solving equation 2.13 for the terminal settling velocity gives:

$$V_{TS} = \frac{\rho_P d^2 g}{18\eta} , d > 1\mu m \text{ and } R_e < 1.0 \tag{2.14}$$

The terminal settling velocity increases when the particle size increases, being proportional to the square of the particle diameter. As expected from the derivation, the settling velocity in the Stokes' region is inversely proportional to the viscosity and does not depend on the density of the gas. Aerosol particles adjust to their terminal settling velocity almost instantly, and V_{TS} is appropriate for characterizing particle motion in most real situations. Equation 2.14 cannot be used for particles smaller than 1.0 μm unless the slip correction factor, covered in the next section, is applied (Moshfegh et al. 2010). The terminal velocity for other kinds of external forces, such as centrifugal force, can be obtained by derivations similar to that given for gravity. In a centrifugal force field, the terminal velocity is given by

$$V_{TC} = \frac{\rho_P d^2 a_C}{18\eta}$$
(2.15)

where, a_c is the centrifugal acceleration at the location of the particle.

For a tangential velocity V_T and the radius of motion R,

$$a_C = \frac{V_T^2}{R}$$
(2.16)

Equation 2.14, is of fundamental importance to aerosol studies. However, in the form given, it is accurate (±10%) only for determining the settling velocity of the standard density particles having diameters of 1.5-75 μm. When slip correction is included, it is accurate for particles as small as 0.001 μm.

In Stokes' law, equation 2.9, the resistance force is directly proportional to the velocity. From this relationship, we can define the particle mobility (B) as a measure of the relative ease of producing a steady motion for an aerosol particle.

$$B = \frac{V}{F_D} = \frac{1}{3\pi\eta d} \quad , d > 1\mu m$$
(2.17)

Mobility is the ratio of the terminal velocity of a particle to the steady force producing that velocity. It has units of m/N.s (cm/dyne. s) and is often called the mechanical mobility to distinguish it from any electrical mobility. The terminal velocity of an aerosol particle is simply the force times mobility; for example,

$$V_{TS} = F_G \cdot B$$
(2.18)

Current research has indicated that an aerosol cloud and individual particle express fairly different settling behaviors. The effect of long-range interparticle with hydrodynamic interactions in the aerosol cloud results in their movement being significantly faster than individual particles with the same magnitude of external forces (Yang et al. 2010).

2.5. Slip Correction Factor

An important assumption of Stokes' law is that the relative velocity of the gas right at the surface of the sphere is zero. This assumption is not met for small particles whose size approaches the mean free path of the gas. Such particles settle faster than one predicted by Stokes' law because there is "slip" at the surface of the particle. At standard conditions, this error becomes significant for particles with a diameter less than 1 μm. In 1910, Cunningham derived a correction factor for Stokes' law to account for the effect of slip. The factor called the *Cunningham correction factor C* was always greater than one and reduced the Stokes drag force by equation 2.19.

$$F_D = \frac{3\pi\eta Vd}{C_C} \tag{2.19}$$

where,

$$C_C = 1 + \frac{2.52\lambda}{d} \tag{2.20}$$

where λ is the mean free path and d is the particle diameter.

Use of the Cunningham correction factor (equation 2.20), extended the range of applications of Stokes' law to particles of 0.1 μm in diameter. This range can be extended to still smaller particles by empirical equations based on experimental measurements of the slip. This factor is called the *slip correction factor* and must be used in the form of equation 2.21 for particles that are less than 0.1 μm in diameter. The slip-corrected form of the terminal settling velocity becomes $R_e < 1.0$ (equation 2.22).

Equation 2.22 is valid for all particle sizes when Re < 1.0 and equation 2.21 is used for

$$C_C = 1 + \frac{\lambda}{d} \left[2.34 + 1.05 exp \left(-0.39 \frac{d}{\lambda} \right) \right] \qquad (2.21)$$

The slip correction factor for a 1.0 μm particle under standard conditions is 1.15; that is, the particle settles 15% faster than predicted by equation 2.14, which is based on the uncorrected form of the Stokes' law. For the particle size of less than 1 μm, the slip increases rapidly as the size decreases, where the Cunningham or slip correction factor must be used (Moshfegh et al. 2009). For accurate work, it should be used for all particles less than 5 or 10 μm. It is commonly stated that a slip correction is necessary for particles as their size approaches the mean free path because "the particles are so small they slip between the molecules" (Hinds 2012). This is incorrect, but a useful way to remember how to apply the slip correction factor (Moshfegh et al. 2010). Slip correction increases as the pressure decreases because the mean free path increases.

$$V_{TS} = \frac{\rho_P d^2 g C_C}{18 \eta} \text{ , for } R_e < 1.0 \qquad (2.22)$$

2.6. Nonspherical Particles

The *equivalent volume diameter* (d_e) is the diameter of a sphere having the same volume as that of the irregular particle. This sphere is called the *equivalent volume sphere.* The equivalent volume diameter can be imagined as the diameter of the sphere that would result if the irregular particle melted to form a droplet.

Dynamic shape factors for particles of various shapes are given in Table 2.2.

Values for the geometric shapes were determined by measuring the settling velocity of geometric models in liquids. For irregular particles, settling velocities were measured indirectly using elutriation devices. Values given in the table are averaged over all orientations, which is the usual situation for the motion of the aerosol particle ($R_e < 0.1$) because of the Brownian motion of the particles. There is an exception for certain streamlined shapes in which the dynamic shape factor is greater than 1.0.

Table 2.2. Dynamic shape factors for particles of various shapes.
(Adapted from Hinds, W. C., John Wiley & Sons, 2012)

Shape	Shape factor	Dynamic shape factor		
Sphere	1.00	Axial ratio		
Cube	1.08	2	5	10
Cylinder*		1.09	1.23	1.43
Straight chain		1.10	1.35	1.68
Three spheres	1.15			
Four spheres	1.17			

*orientation average

This means that non-spherical particles settle more slowly than their equivalent volume spheres (Mand and Rosendahl 2010).

$$X = \frac{F_D}{3\pi\eta V d_e} \tag{2.23}$$

$$F_D = 3\pi\eta V d_e X \tag{2.24}$$

2.7. Aerodynamic Diameter

An equivalent diameter (d_e) that has found wide applications in aerosol technology is the *aerodynamic diameter d_a*. This is defined as the diameter of a spherical particle with a density of 1 g/cm^3 that has the same settling velocity. The aerodynamic diameter standardizes for a spherical shape and unit density (1 g/cm^3).

A related equivalent diameter is the *Stokes diameter d_{st}* which is the diameter of a sphere that has the same density and settling velocity as the particle.

Equation 2.25 can be written in terms of these diameters that neglects any slip correction,

$$V_{TS} = \frac{\rho_P d_e^2 g}{18\eta X} \tag{2.25}$$

where, ρ_0 is the standard particle density, 1.0 g/cm^3.

The aerodynamic diameter can be defined as the diameter of a water droplet that will have the same aerodynamic properties as the particle. If a particle has an aerodynamic diameter of 1 μm, it behaves in an aerodynamic sense like a 1 μm water droplet regardless of its shape, density or physical size. Furthermore, it is aerodynamically indistinguishable from other particles of different size, shape, and density having aerodynamic diameters of 1 μm. The Stokes' diameter is usually defined in terms of the normal density of the bulk material of the particle ρ_b. This definition avoids the problem of defining the true density of the particle which may be less than ρ_b due to porosity, occlusions or an agglomerated structure.

$$V_{TS} = \frac{\rho_P d_e^2 g}{18\eta X} = \frac{\rho_0 d_a^2 g}{18\eta} = \frac{\rho_b d_{st}^2 g}{18\eta} \tag{2.26}$$

2.8. Settling at High Reynolds Numbers

For particle motion in the Stokes region, the settling velocity can be determined explicitly if the particle diameter and density are known; the diameter can be found if the velocity is known. However, for particle motion with Re > 1.0, this is not the case.

References

Dechraksa, Janwit, Tan Suwandecha, Kittinan Maliwan, and Teerapol Srichana. 2014. "The comparison of fluid dynamics parameters in an Andersen cascade impactor equipped with and without a preseparator." *AAPS PharmSciTech* 15 (3):792-801. doi: 10.1208/s12249-014-0102-2.

Hinds, William C. 2012. *Aerosol Technology: Properties, Behavior, and Measurement of Airborne Particles*. 2nd ed. Noboken, NJ: John Wiley & Sons, Inc.

Ma, Baoshun, and Chantal Darquenne. 2011. "Aerosol deposition characteristics in distal acinar airways under cyclic breathing conditions." *Journal of Applied Physiology* 110 (5):1271-1282. doi: 10.1152/jappl physiol.00735.2010.

Mand, Matthias, and Lasse Rosendahl. 2010. "On the motion of non-spherical particles at high Reynolds number." *Powder Technology* 202:1-13.

Moshfegh, Abouzar, Mehrzad Shams, Goodarz Ahmadi, and Reza Ebrahimi. 2009. "A novel surface-slip correction for microparticles motion." *Colloids and Surfaces A: Physicochemical and Engineering Aspects* 345:112-120.

Moshfegh, Abouzar, Mehrzad Shams, Goodarz Ahmadi, and Reza Ebrahimi. 2010. "A new expression for spherical aerosol drag in slip flow regime." *Journal of Aerosol Science* 41:384-400.

Nicolaou, Laura, and Tamer A. Zaki. 2013. "Direct numerical simulations of flow in realistic mouth–throat geometries." *Journal of Aerosol Science* 57:71-87. doi: 10.1016/j.jaerosci.2012.10.003.

Theerachaisupakij, Woraporn, Shuji Matsusaka, Y. Akashi, and Hiroaki Masuda. 2002. "Reentrainment of deposited particles by drag and aerosol collision." *Journal of Aerosol Science* 34:261-274.

Yang, Wei, Keat Theng Chow, Bo Lang, Nathan P. Wiederhold, Keith P. Johnston, and Robert O. Williams. 2010. "In vitro characterization and pharmacokinetics in mice following pulmonary delivery of itraconazole as cyclodextrin solubilized solution." *European Journal of Pharmaceutical Sciences* 39 (5):336-347. doi: 10.1016/j.ejps.2010.01.001.

Chapter 3

Forces and Interactions

3.1. Introduction

The terminal velocity of a particle moving in the Stokes region is directly proportional to the net external force F acting on the particle. Here, 'external force' means a force acting remotely on a particle, such as gravity, centrifugal or electrostatic forces. The drag force is not considered an external force. The constant of proportionality is the mechanical mobility B that is defined by an Equation 3.1.

$$V_{TS} = BF \qquad (3.1)$$

When the external force is the force of gravity, equation 3.1 becomes

$$V_{TS} = BF_G = Bmg \qquad (3.2)$$

The product of particle mass and mobility, mB, frequently occurs in aerosol mechanics and it is a useful quantity for the analysis of the complex motion of a particle. This quantity is called the *relaxation time* of the particle and is given the symbol τ.

The term "relaxation time" is used because it characterizes the time required for a particle to adjust or "relax" its velocity to a new set of force conditions. The relaxation time is analogous to a characteristic acceleration time for a moving object. It depends only on the mass and mobility of the particle and is not affected by the nature or magnitude of the external forces acting on the particle. Although it is useful to think of the relaxation time as a particle property, it includes viscosity and slip correction and is thus affected by the temperature and pressure of the surrounding gas (Moshfegh et al. 2010, 2009). The use of relaxation time as defined by equation 3.2 is restricted to particle motion in the Stokes region, where $R_e < 1$. Relaxation time increases rapidly with particle size because it is proportional to the square of the diameter as described in equation 3.3.

$$\tau = mB = \rho_p \frac{\pi}{6} d^3 \left(\frac{C_c}{3\pi\eta d} \right) = \frac{\rho_p d^2 C_c}{18\eta} = \frac{\rho_0 d_a^2 C_c}{18\eta} \tag{3.3}$$

Relaxation time can be used to simplify the calculation of a particle's terminal settling velocity. Substituting τ in equation 3.2 gives

$$V_{TS} = \tau g \tag{3.4}$$

The terminal velocity of a particle is simply the product of τ and the acceleration caused by an external force. For any constant external force F acting on a particle of mass m, the terminal velocity is

$$\sum F = m \frac{dV(t)}{dt} = ma(t) \tag{3.5}$$

The equations for a particle's terminal settling velocity that are derived in the previous chapter ignore the acceleration of the particle considering only the equilibrium condition when the forces acting on the particle are balanced and the velocity of the particle is constant. We now consider the acceleration of a particle that is released with zero initial velocity in still air. The particle quickly reaches its terminal settling velocity, and we wish to know how long that takes and the nature of the acceleration process. Newton's second law of motion must hold at every instant during the acceleration process.

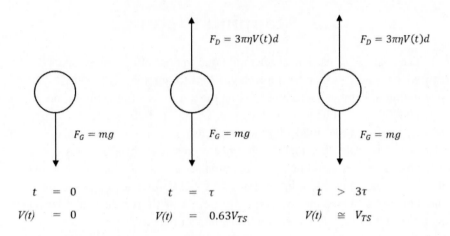

Figure 3.1. Acceleration of a particle in still air.

$$F_G - F_D = mg - 3\pi\eta V(t)d = m\frac{dV(t)}{dt} \tag{3.6}$$

Multiplying both sides of equation 3.6 by the particle mobility B gives equation 3.7.

Replacing τg with V_{TS} and rearranging, we obtain

$$mBg - 3\pi\eta V(t)Bd = mB\frac{dV(t)}{dt} \tag{3.7}$$

$$\tau g - V(t) = \tau\frac{dV(t)}{dt} \tag{3.8}$$

$$\int_0^t \frac{dt}{\tau} = \int_0^{V(t)} \frac{dV(t)}{V_{TS} - V(t)} \tag{3.9}$$

$$\frac{t}{\tau} = -\ln[V_{TS} - V(t)] + \ln V_{TS} \tag{3.10}$$

$$e^{-t/\tau} = \frac{V_{TS} - V(t)}{V_{TS}} \tag{3.11}$$

3.2. Stopping Distance

The analysis of particle acceleration due to constant external forces can be carried one step further by replacing *V(t)* in equation 3.11 with *dx/dt* and integrating to get the displacement along the x-axis as a function of time, *x(t):*

The Stokes number is defined in equation 3.12 where the *stopping distance* (S) is the total distance traveled or the inertial range. On a displacement scale, the stopping distance represents a measure of a particle's effective initial momentum which is diminished to zero by air friction over a distance equal to the stopping distance. As τ is defined as the product of *mB,* the stopping distance can be defined in terms of the product of a particle's mobility and its initial momentum. D_j is the jet diameter.

In a mathematical sense, it will take an infinite time for a particle to travel its entire stopping distance, but in a practical sense, the particle travels 95% of that distance very rapidly in a time equal to 3 τ. The stopping distance represents the ultimate distance a particle will travel in still air if the external force acting on the particle is suddenly turned off, as might be the case for an electrical force. A more important use of the stopping distance is for a particle moving with an airstream that is abruptly turned 90°. In this case, the stopping distance represents the distance the particle continues to travel in its original direction and thus can be thought as a measure of the "persistence" of the particle. The preceding discussion of stopping distance assumes that the entire motion of a particle takes place within the Stokes region. The stopping distance is the most important for large particles with high velocities that frequently have motion, at least initially outside the Stokes region. This situation is very difficult to analyze.

The situation is more complicated for flow around an obstacle. Very small particles with negligible inertia will follow the gas streamlines perfectly. Large and heavy particles will tend to continue in a straight line, regardless of what the gas flow does. The particles of interest are those whose motion lies between these extremes.

To analyze this type of motion, one first defines the flow field and the pattern of streamlines for the gas flow around the obstacle. This can be a difficult fluid mechanics problem. Once the flow field is defined, the velocity and direction of the flow are known for every point near the obstacle. The actual particle trajectory is determined as it proceeds through the flow field. The analysis can be done only for very simple geometries, such as flow around a spherical or cylindrical obstacle. With more complicated shapes, it can be done numerically by following a series of incremental steps through the flow field. The forces on the particles are assumed to be constant during each step and are re-evaluated for each step. Usually, this analysis is done for a large number of starting positions of the particle relative to the obstacle.

3.3. Stokes Number

Curvilinear motion is characterized by a dimensionless number called the *Stokes number* (Stk). It is the ratio of the stopping distance of a particle (S) to a characteristic dimension of the obstacle (d_c). For example, for a flow perpendicular to a cylinder of diameter d_c, the Stokes number is an equation 3.12.

$$Stk = \frac{S}{d_c} = \frac{\tau U_0}{d_c}, \qquad \text{for R}_e < 1.0 \tag{3.12}$$

Where, U_o is the undisturbed air velocity well away from the cylinder and $R_{eo} = \rho_g \, d_p U_o / \eta$ when $R_e > 1.0$. The Stokes number is also the ratio of the particle relaxation time to the transit time past an obstacle or the ratio of the time τ it takes for a particle to adjust to the time $d_c U$ available for adjustment. When Stk >> 1, particles continue moving in a straight line when the gas turns; when Stk << 1, particles follow the gas streamlines perfectly. Because the characteristic dimension d_c in equation 3.12 can be defined differently for different applications, the definition of Stokes number may be application specific.

For a geometrically similar particle motion to occur around different-sized cylinders, two conditions must be met: (1) the flow Reynolds numbers for the two situations must be equal, and (2) the Stokes numbers must be equal. Equality of the Reynolds numbers ensures that the gas flows are similar, and the equality of the Stokes numbers ensures that the particle motion in the flow fields is also similar. The Stokes number is the ratio of a particle's "persistence" to the size of the obstacle.

As the Stokes number approaches zero, particles track the streamlines perfectly. As the Stokes number increases, the particles resist changing their direction when the gas streamlines change directions. The Stokes number is used to characterize the *inertial impaction* which is the inertial transfer of particles onto surfaces that is described in the next section.

The concept of an inertial impaction has evolved into a virtual impactor. The airborne particles do not physically collide with a collection plate as occurs in a conventional impactor in which the particles are selectively filtered by the airflow. The virtual impactor was designed to split the airflow into a major and minor flow (Marple and Olson 2011). The minor flow mimics the impaction plate in a conventional impactor (Lee et al. 2014). It captures the particles that are larger than the cut-off size along with the flow. The major flow separates particles that are smaller than the cut-off of the virtual impactor. Recently, a ring-shaped nozzle was developed as a novel aerosol impactor (Son et al. 2015). The collection efficiency curve and Stk_{50} of an impactor with an orifice become respectively steeper and smaller than an impactor without an orifice.

3.4. Inertial Impaction

Impaction is a special case of curvilinear motion of aerosol particles. As a result of its importance, impaction has been analyzed theoretically and experimentally more than any other aerosol separation process (Erdal and Esmen 1990). In the first half of this century, impaction was a common method for collecting dust for the evaluation of occupational environments. Since the 1960s, cascade impactor instruments based on impaction have been used extensively for the measurement of particle size distributions by mass.

All inertial impactors operate on the same principle. An aerosol is passed through a nozzle and the output stream (jet) directed against a flat plate (Figure 3.2). The flat plate is called an *impaction plate* which deflects the flow abruptly in a 90° bend in the streamlines. Particles whose inertia exceeds a certain value are unable to follow the streamlines and will impact on the plate.

It is assumed that larger particles will stick to the surface if they hit whereas the smaller particles will remain airborne, follow the streamlines and flow out of the impactor. Thus, an impactor separates aerosol particles into two size ranges; particles larger than a certain aerodynamic size are removed from the airstream and those smaller than that size remains in the airstream.

Impactor theory seeks to explain the shape of the curve of the collection efficiency versus the particle size (Figure 3.3). The parameter that governs the collection efficiency is the Stokes number or the impaction parameter which is defined for an impactor as the ratio of the particle stopping distance at the average nozzle exit velocity U to the jet radius $D_j/2$.

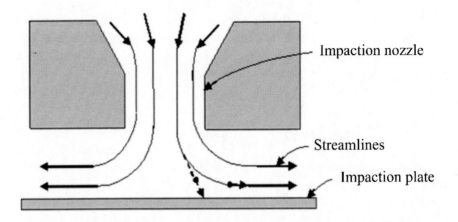

Figure 3.2. Cross-sectional view of an impactor. (Adapted from Hinds, W. C., John Wiley & Sons, 2012).

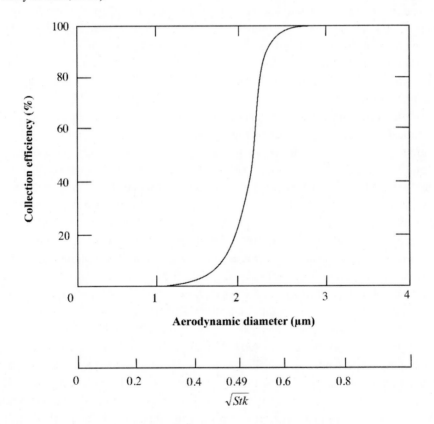

Figure 3.3. Typical impactor efficiency.

This Stokes number is slightly different from equation 3.12, being defined in terms of the nozzle radius $D_j/2$ rather than a characteristic dimension of an obstacle. For an impactor with a rectangular nozzle, the jet half-width should be used in place of the jet radius in equation 3.13.

$$Stk = \frac{\tau U}{D_j / 2} = \frac{\rho_p d_p^2 U C_c}{9\eta D_j} \qquad (3.13)$$

Although the collection efficiency is a function of the Stokes number, there is no simple relationship between the impactor collection efficiency and the Stokes number. Theoretical determination of the characteristic efficiency curve for an impactor requires numerical analysis using a computer (Abouali, Saadabadi, and Emdad 2011). First, the pattern of streamlines in the vicinity of the jet is determined by solving the Navier-Stokes equations for a particular impactor geometry (Dechraksa et al. 2014). Then, for a given particle size, particle trajectories are determined for each that enters the streamline. The efficiency for that particle size is determined by the fraction of the trajectories that intercept the impaction plate. This process is repeated for many particle sizes in order to generate the characteristic impactor efficiency curve such as the one shown in Figure 3.3.

The collection efficiency curves for the impactors are often plotted in a general form as efficiency versus the square root of the Stokes number ($Stk^{0.5}$) which is directly proportional to the particle size. Experimental calibration requires efficient measurements made with a series of monodisperse aerosols (Srichana, Martin, and Marriott 1998). However, this needs to be done at least once for each impactor design, because all geometrically similar impactors that meet the recommended design criteria, given later, will have the same collection efficiency when operated at the same Stokes number. The *simplified* analysis serves to illustrate the process of impaction and the importance of the relevant parameters. It is necessary to make the simplifying assumption that the flow velocity is uniform in the jet and the streamlines are arcs of a circle with their centers at A. Figure 3.4 illustrates a cross-sectional view of a rectangular jet impactor. Because of the symmetry, only one-half of the impactor needs to be considered. A particle exiting the nozzle along a streamline experiences a centrifugal force causing it to move toward the impaction plate. If these departures are slight, as will be the case for the limiting condition that separates impaction from no impaction, the particle will depart from its original streamline with a constant radial velocity (V_r) while traversing the curved part of the streamline. This velocity is given by

$$V_r = \tau a_r = \frac{\tau U^2}{r} \tag{3.14}$$

where, r is the radius of curvature of the streamline.

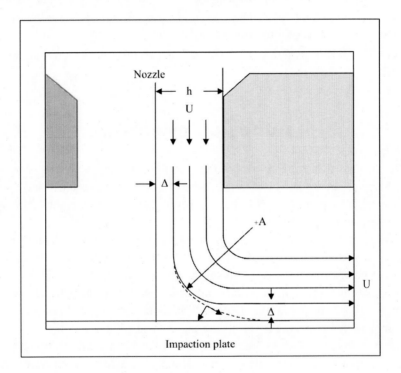

Figure 3.4. Simplified impactor model. (Adapted from Hinds, W. C., John Wiley & Sons, 2012).

3.5. Straight-Line Acceleration and Curvilinear Particle Motion

If the velocity remains constant in the curved-streamline region, the total radial displacement of the particle from its original streamline is the product of its radial velocity and the time required to traverse the curved portion (quarter circle) of the streamline.

At the end of the quarter circle, each particle will have moved a distance Δ from its original streamline in the direction of the impaction surface. Any particle passing through the nozzle within a distance Δ of the jet centerline will end up impacting on the plate (Figure 3.4). Particles located more than a distance Δ from the centerline will be shifted from their original streamlines, but not enough to reach the impaction surface. Because Figure 3.4 is a transverse section of a rectangular nozzle, the impaction efficiency (E_I) the fraction of entering particles collected is equal to the ratio of the lengths Δ and h.

3.6. Adhesion of Particles

Aerosol particles attach firmly to any surface they contact. This is one of the characteristics that distinguish them from gas molecules and from millimeter-sized particles. Whenever aerosol particles contact one another, they adhere and form agglomerates.

Filtration and other particle collection methods rely on the adhesion of particles to surfaces. The adhesive forces on micrometer-sized particles exceed other common forces by orders of magnitude.

Despite its importance, particle adhesion is poorly understood and its description is partly qualitative. Because it is such a complicated phenomenon, no complete theory accounts for all the factors that influence adhesion. Much of the experimental work on particle adhesion has been conducted with ideal surfaces under special conditions, such as a high vacuum, which have little relevance to real surfaces of practical interest.

3.7. Adhesive Forces

The main adhesive forces are the van der Waals force, the electrostatic force and the force arising from the surface tension of adsorbed liquid films. All of these forces are affected by the material shape, the surface roughness and the size of the particle, the material roughness and the contamination of the surface, the relative humidity, temperature, the duration of the contact, and the initial contact velocity (Cheng, Dunn, and Brach 2002, Karner, Littringer, and Urbanetz 2014).

First, consider the theoretical description of the adhesive forces. The most important forces are the London-van der Waals forces which are the long-range attractive forces that exist between molecules. These forces are long range in comparison to chemical bonds which are called short-range forces. Because of the shielding effects of the adsorbed layers of water and organic molecules, chemical bonds are not important for the adhesion of aerosol particles under ambient conditions. The van der Waals forces arise because of the random movement of the electrons in any material that creates momentary areas of concentrated charge called dipoles. At any instant, these dipoles induce complementary dipoles in neighboring materials which in turn produce attractive forces (Figure 3.5). Van der Waals forces decrease rapidly with the separation distance between the surfaces; consequently, their influence extends only a few molecular diameters away from a surface.

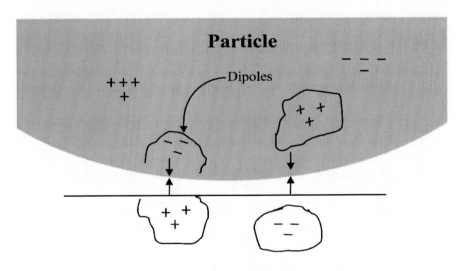

Figure 3.5 van der Waals adhesive forces.

At a submicroscopic level, most surfaces are irregular with peaks called asperities, and valleys (Figure 3.6). At least initially, contact between a particle and a surface occurs only at a few asperities. Most of the material is separated by an average distance x that depends on the scale of surface roughness (Figure 3.6). For smooth surfaces, this distance is usually assumed to be 0.4 nm which is about the size of the molecules involved.

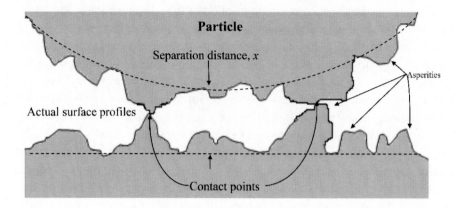

Figure 3.6. Submicroscopic surface contact geometry.

The net effect of the van der Waals forces is determined by integrating the forces between all pairs of molecules of a spherical particle near a flat surface. The resulting adhesive force between the particle and a plane surface is

$$F = \frac{Ad}{12x^2}$$
(3.15)

where, A is the Hamaker constant which depends on the materials involved and ranges from 6×10^{-20} to 150×10^{-20} J for common materials. Equation 3.15 applies to hard materials with negligible flattening in the contact area. After the initial particle contact, the van der Waals and electrostatic forces gradually deform the asperities to reduce the separation distance and increase the contact area until the attractive forces balance the forces resisting deformation. The deformation process may take as long as a few hours. The hardness of the materials involved controls the size of the ultimate area of contact and therefore the strength of the adhesive force.

Most particles of size 0.1 μm or larger carry some small net charge q which induces an equal and opposite charge on the surface. Coulomb's law is one basis to describe the electrostatic attraction of charged particles. The magnitude of the electrostatic force is defined by two factors that are the amount of the charges that particles carry and the distance between the charged particles (Jiang, Hansen, and Raymond 2010). This gives an attractive electrostatic force of

$$F_E = \frac{K_E q^2}{x_q^2} \tag{3.16}$$

where, K_E is a constant of proportionality and x_q is the separation distance of opposite charges which may be different from the separation distance between the surfaces.

Particles of insulating material at low humidities retain their charge and are held to surfaces by the electrostatic force. The electrostatic charges during the aerosolization ranged from 0.1 to 0.3 nC/mg from a 30–90 LPM flow rate. Thus, electrostatic effect can be omitted and it does not have any significant role in the aerosolization performance (Suwandecha et al. 2014). The equilibrium charge carried by particles larger than 0.1 μm is approximately proportional to $\sqrt{d}$, so the electrostatic adhesion force is also proportional to the first power of the particle diameter.

Under normal conditions, most materials have adsorbed liquid molecules on their surface. An attractive force between a particle and a surface is created by the surface tension of the liquid drawn into the capillary space at the point of contact (Figure 3.7). For relative humidities greater than 90% and ideal smooth surfaces, this force is

$$F_S = 2\pi\gamma d \tag{3.17}$$

where, γ is the surface tension of the liquid. For real surfaces at lower relative humidities, the force depends on the curvature of the asperities at the points of contact and not on the particle diameter. This curvature varies greatly from particle to particle and gives rise to a distribution of adhesive forces for the same sized particles.

The three adhesive forces just discussed are all proportional to the first power of the particle diameter, and this is the form of most empirical expressions for an adhesive force. Except for highly charged particles, van der Waals and surface tension forces are greater than electrostatic forces.

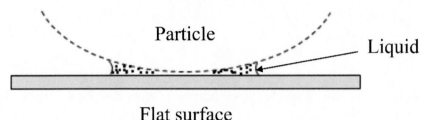

Flat surface

Figure 3.7. Adhesive forces due to a liquid film.

Experimental measurements of adhesive forces are made by determining the force required to separate a particle from a surface. They may be direct measurements using a centrifugal force (Ahmad, Ungphaiboon, and Srichana 2015), or the indirect measurements using vibration or air currents to remove the particles. For hard materials and clean surfaces a useful empirical expression for the adhesive force, based on direct measurement of glass and quartz particles (> 20 μm) at 25°C is given in Newtons for force, in meters for the particle diameter and in percent for relative humidity (%RH).

3.8. Detachment of Particles

The force required to detach particles from a surface can be measured by subjecting the particles to a centrifugal force normal to the surface in a centrifuge and determining the rotational speed required to detach the particles. These experiments yield a distribution of forces required to remove monodisperse particles from a surface. About 10 times as much force is required to remove 98% of the particles as that required for 50% removal (Ahmad, Ungphaiboon, and Srichana 2015). Particles can also be removed by air currents directed at the surface.

Adhesive forces are proportional to d, while removal forces are proportional to d^3 for gravitational, vibrational and centrifugal forces, and d^2 for air currents. These relationships indicate that as the particle size decreases, it becomes more difficult to remove particles from surfaces. This fact agrees without intuition that large, visible particles such as grains of sand can be removed by shaking or air currents, but smaller ones cannot, although they may be removed by washing. The important point is that the adhesive force on a particle size of less than 10 μm is much greater than other forces on such a particle (Begat et al. 2004).

While individual particles of less than 10 μm are not likely to be removed by common forces, a thick layer of such particles may be easily dislodged in large chunks (0.1-10 mm). The particles adhere tightly to each other and form large agglomerates that can be easily blown or shaken from the surface.

3.9. Resuspension

Closely related to adhesion and detachment of particles is the process of *resuspension* which can be defined as the detachment of a particle from a surface and its transport away from the surface (Selvam et al. 2010). Resuspension may occur as a result of air jets, mechanical forces, impaction of other particles or electrostatic forces. Re-entrainment or *blow-off,* a more specific term, refers to resuspension by a jet of air. As with other aspects of adhesion, we understand the nature of the process but are unable to predict reliably when resuspension will occur. Re-entrainment of deposited particles may occur by drag and aerosol collision (Theerachaisupakij et al. 2002).

Unlike static adhesion, described in the preceding sections, resuspension may involve rolling or sliding of the particle before it becomes airborne. Forces required to remove a particle under these circumstances are approximately 1% less than those required for static detachment in a centrifuge. To analyze re-entrainment by an air jet or by airflow in a tube, we consider two cases: individual particles on a surface (a sparse monolayer) and an adhering dust layer wherein particles contact each other. While it is relatively easy to determine the jet or duct velocity and whether a particle has been removed, it is difficult to determine the air velocity and resulting drag force on a particle adhering to a surface.

Re-entrainment is a stochastic process in which a given condition of air velocity permits one to estimate only the fraction of particles of a given size that will be removed from a surface. The larger the particle and greater the air velocity, the greater the probability of re-entrainment.

For the usual case of a turbulent airstream, there is a thin layer of laminar airflow at the surface called the *boundary layer* or *laminar sublayer.* Particles smaller than this layer are partially protected from re-entrainment by being submerged in the boundary layer. Re-entrainment of particles submerged in the boundary layer occurs as a result of occasional bursts of turbulent eddies penetrating through the boundary layer to detach particles. Thus, such re-entrainment is time dependent.

The situation is different if a layer of particles is present on a surface. Two processes may occur. First, particles may be re-entrained from the top surface of the layer as individual particles or small clusters. This is called *erosion.* Alternatively, a whole section of the layer can be re-entrained in a process called denudation. The occurrence of such process depends on the relative strength of the adhesive forces between the particles and between the particles and the surface. Erosion increases with the duration of exposure to an air jet, while denudation is complete in less than a second.

3.10. Particle Bounce

When a solid particle contacts a surface at a low velocity that is less than a few m/s the particle loses its kinetic energy by deforming itself and the surface. The greater the velocity, the greater the deformation and better the adhesion. At high velocities, part of the kinetic energy is dissipated in the deformation process (plastic deformation) and part is converted elastically to the kinetic energy of rebound (Wall et al. 1990). If the rebound energy exceeds the adhesion forces, a particle will bounce away from the surface. Bouncing can occur in particle sizes that would adhere tightly in a static situation; it does not occur for droplets or easily deformed materials such as tar. Maximum rebound velocities occur at intermediate approach velocities.

The problem of particle bounce has been studied for solid particle collection in impactors and fibrous filters. The harder the particle material, the larger the particle or the greater its velocity, a bounce will more occur, although surface roughness plays a significant role. Coating the surfaces with oil or grease increases the adhesion energy, the deformation, and the dissipative energy greatly reduces the problem of bounce (Srichana, Martin, and Marriott 1998, 2000).

There are two approaches to define the conditions at which bounce will occur. One approach defines the limiting adhesion or kinetic energy and the other defines a critical velocity V_c for which bounce will occur if that velocity is exceeded.

$$V_c = \frac{\beta}{d_a} \tag{3.18}$$

The latter forms equation 3.18 where β is a constant that depends on the materials used and the geometry of the situation. For example, $\beta = 2 \times 10^{-6}$ m^2/s defines an upper limit of velocity for which bounce will *not* occur on uncoated metal impaction plates. Measurements of V_c by Wall et al. (1990) for ammonium fluorescein particles impacting four target materials gave β values that ranged from 7.4×10^{-6} to 2.9×10^{-5}.

The kinetic energy (KE_b) required for bounce to occur when a particle collides with a surface is given by Dahneke (1971) as

$$KE_b = \frac{d_p A\left(1 - e^2\right)}{2xe^2} \tag{3.19}$$

where, x is the separation distance, defined previously, A is the Hamaker constant, and e is the coefficient of restitution which is equal to the ratio of the rebound velocity to the approach velocity. Representative values for e range from 0.73 to 0.81 (Wall et al. 1990). A and e depend only on the particle material and its surface.

In practice, one relies on the experimental determination of these constants. A regression by Ellenbecker, Leith, and Price (1980) gives the probability of bounce (P_b) for irregular fly ash particles with CMD = 0.14 μm versus their approach kinetic energy in J.

For cgs units, KE is in ergs and 0.000224 is replaced by 0.00958. Equation (3.20) agrees reasonably well with measurements made by Suwandecha, Wongpoowarak, and Srichana (2016). The equation gives 0 and 50% probability of bounce at KEs of 2×10^{-16} and 4×10^{-15} J, respectively. These values correspond to the approach velocities of 0.03 m/s and 0.12 m/s for 10 μm particles of standard density.

$$P_b = 1 - 0.000224\left(KE\right)^{-0.233} \tag{3.20}$$

3.11. Diffusion Coefficient

Brownian motion is the random wiggling motion of an aerosol particle in the still air caused by random variations in the relentless bombardment of gas molecules against the particle. *Diffusion* of aerosol particles is the *net* transport of these particles in a concentration gradient. This transport is always from a region of higher concentration to a region of lower concentration. Both processes are characterized by the particle diffusion coefficient D. The larger the value of D, the more vigorous the Brownian motion and more rapid the mass transfer in a concentration gradient. The diffusion coefficient is the constant of proportionality that relates the flux J of aerosol particles (the net number of particles traveling through unit cross section each second) to the concentration gradient dn/dx. This relationship is called *Fick's first law of diffusion.* In the absence of any external forces, Fick's law is

$$J = -D\,dn/dx \qquad\qquad (3.21)$$

The diffusion coefficient of an aerosol particle can be expressed in terms of the particle properties by the Stokes-Einstein derivation. In this derivation, the diffusion force on the particles that causes their net motion down the concentration gradient, is equated to the force exerted by the gas resisting the motion of the particles.

Einstein (1905) showed that (1) the observable Brownian motion of an aerosol particle is equivalent to that of a giant gas molecule; (2) the kinetic energy of an aerosol particle undergoing Brownian motion is the same as that of the gas molecules within which it is suspended ($KE = 3/2kT$); (3) the diffusion force on a particle is the net osmotic pressure force on that particle.

Osmotic pressure is best understood by considering dissolved molecules in liquids. A semipermeable membrane permits liquid molecules to pass through it unimpeded but prevents dissolved molecules from passing through. The membrane is free to slide to the left or right. If it is moved to a given position toward the left, it must be applied to hold it in place. This force equals the net osmotic pressure force acting to the right. The latter can be thought of as a pressure created by the high concentration of dissolved molecules on the left side of the membrane or pressure caused by the liquid trying to get to the region of low liquid concentration (due to the high concentration of dissolved molecules) and equalize the concentration. The force is directly proportional to the difference in concentrations on either side of the membrane. These concepts apply equally well to particles suspended in gasses and to dissolved molecules in liquids.

References

Abouali, Omid, Saeideh Saadabadi, and Homayoon Emdad. 2011. "Numerical investigation of the flow field and cut-off characteristics of supersonic/hypersonic impactors." *Journal of Aerosol Science* 42 (2):65-77. doi: 10.1016/j.jaerosci.2010.11.006.

Ahmad, Md Iftekhar, Suwipa Ungphaiboon, and Teerapol Srichana. 2015. "The development of dimple-shaped chitosan carrier for ethambutol dihydrochloride dry powder inhaler." *Drug Development and Industrial Pharmacy* 41 (5):791-800. doi: 10.3109/03639045.2014.903493.

Begat, Philippe, David A. V. Morton, John N. Staniforth, and Robert Price. 2004. "The cohesive-adhesive balances in dry powder inhaler formulations II: Influence on fine particle delivery characteristics." *Pharmaceutical Research* 21 (10):1826-1834.

Cheng, W., Patrick F. Dunn, and Raymond M. Brach. 2002. "Surface roughness effects on microparticle adhesion." *The Journal of Adhesion* 78 (11):929-965

Dahneke, Barton. 1971. "The capture of aerosol particles by surfaces." *Journal of Colloid and Interface Science* 37 (2):342-353.

Dechraksa, Janwit, Tan Suwandecha, Kittinan Maliwan, and Teerapol Srichana. 2014. "The comparison of fluid dynamics parameters in an Andersen cascade impactor equipped with and without a preseparator." *AAPS PharmSciTech* 15 (3):792-801. doi: 10.1208/s12249-014-0102-2.

Einstein, Albert. 1905. "On the movement of small particles suspended in stationary liquids required by the molecular-kinetic theory of heat." *Annalen der Physik* 17:549-560.

Ellenbecker, Michael J., David Leith, and John M. Price. 1980. "Impaction and particle bounce at high Stokes numbers." *Journal of the Air Pollution Control Association* 30 (11):1224-1227. doi: 10.1080/00022470. 1980.10465173.

Erdal, Serap, and Nurtan A. Esmen. 1990. "The curvilinear motion of coarse particles: New thoughts on theory and applications." *Journal of Aerosol Science* 21 (3):431-440. doi: 10.1016/0021-8502(90)90071-5.

Hinds, William C. 2012. *Aerosol Technology: Properties, Behavior, and Measurement of Airborne Particles*: John Wiley & Sons.

Jiang, Lu, Nordsiek Hansen, and A. Shaw Raymond. 2010. "Clustering of settling charged particles in turbulence: theory and experiments." *New Journal of Physics* 12 (12):123030.

Karner, Stefan, Eva Maria Littringer, and Nora Anne Urbanetz. 2014. "Triboelectrics: The influence of particle surface roughness and shape on charge acquisition during aerosolization and the DPI performance." *Powder Technology* 262:22-29. doi: 10.1016/j.powtec.2014.04.025.

Lee, Handol, Dae-Hyeon Jo, Won-Geun Kim, Se-Jin Yook, and Kang-Ho Ahn. 2014. "Effect of an orifice on collection efficiency and wall loss of a slit virtual impactor." *Aerosol Science and Technology* 48 (2):121-127. doi: 10.1080/02786826.2013.862333.

Marple, Virgil A., and Bernard A. Olson. 2011. "History of Virtual Impactors." In *Aerosol Science and Technology: History and Reviews*, edited by David S. Ensor. Reston, VA: RTI Press.

Moshfegh, Abouzar, Mehrzad Shams, Goodarz Ahmadi, and Reza Ebrahimi. 2009. "A novel surface-slip correction for microparticles motion." *Colloids and Surfaces A: Physicochemical and Engineering Aspects* 345:112-120.

Moshfegh, Abouzar, Mehrzad Shams, Goodarz Ahmadi, and Reza Ebrahimi. 2010. "A new expression for spherical aerosol drag in slip flow regime." *Journal of Aerosol Science* 41:384-400.

Selvam, Parthiban, Steve Marek, C. Randall Truman, Doug McNair, and Hugh D. C. Smyth. 2010. "Micronized drug adhesion and detachment from surfaces: Effect of loading conditions." *Aerosol Science and Technology* 45 (1):81-87. doi: 10.1080/02786826.2010.522628.

Son, Minsoo, Seungho Lim, Giwoon Sung, Taesung Kim, Yeonchul Ha, Kibong Choi, and Weon Gyu Shin. 2015. "Development of a novel aerosol impactor utilizing inward flow from a ring-shaped nozzle." *Journal of Aerosol Science* 85:1-9. doi: 10.1016/j.jaerosci.2015.02.004.

Srichana, Teerapol, Gary P. Martin, and Christopher M. Marriott. 2000. "A human oral-throat cast integrated with a twin-stage impinger for evaluation of dry powder inhalers." *Journal of Pharmacy and Pharmacology* 52 (7):771-778.

Srichana, Teerapol, Gary P. Martin, and Christopher Marriott. 1998. "Calibration method for the Andersen cascade impactor." *Journal of Aerosol Science* 29 (SUPPL.2):S761-S762.

Suwandecha, Tan, Wibul Wongpoowarak, Kittinan Maliwan, and Teerapol Srichana. 2014. "Effect of turbulent kinetic energy on dry powder inhaler performance." *Powder Technology* 267:381-391. doi: 10.1016/j.powtec.2014.07.044.

Suwandecha, Tan, Wibul Wongpoowarak, and Teerapol Srichana. 2016. "Computer-aided design of dry powder inhalers using computational fluid dynamics to assess performance." *Pharmaceutical Development and Technology* 21 (1):54-60. doi: 10.3109/10837450.2014.965325.

Theerachaisupakij, Woraporn, Shuji Matsusaka, Y. Akashi, and Hiroaki Masuda. 2002. "Reentrainment of deposited particles by drag and aerosol collision." *Journal of Aerosol Science* 34:261-274.

Wall, Stephen, Walter John, Hwa-Chi Wang, and Simon L. Goren. 1990. "Measurements of kinetic energy loss for particles impacting surfaces." *Aerosol Science and Technology* 12 (4):926-946. doi: 10.1080/02786829008959404.

Chapter 4

Formulation Design and Production Technology in Dry Powder Inhalers

4.1. Introduction

Aerosol inhalation is a preferred route for drug delivery to the respiratory tract since it confers many distinct advantages over delivery via other routes. The medication is directly delivered to the desired region of the airway and thus the inhalation of an antibiotic for the treatment of lung infection provides an action without wastage through the systemic circulation. Aerosol inhalation also allows for a rapid and predictable onset of action. For instance, after an oral dose of salbutamol, it may take two to three hours before the peak plasma concentration of the drug is achieved and the maximum therapeutic effect obtained, while the corresponding time after administration of an inhaled dose may be only 15 to 30 min (Srichana, Suedee, and Reanmongkol 2001). The first-pass effect is avoided, and even though pulmonary tissues contain a highly developed cytochrome P-450 system capable of inactivating certain drugs, the concentration of cytochrome P-450 present in pulmonary tissues is much less than in the liver. Lower doses can be administered via the respiratory tract, in comparison to other routes. This minimizes any unwanted side effects. For example, an inhaled dose of 100 μg salbutamol sulfate is bioequivalent to 4 mg of the same drug taken orally. Thus, there is a potential for considerable cost savings. Aerosol inhalation can be employed as an alternative route to avoid drug interaction when two or more medications are used concurrently. Conversely, this route does have some disadvantages such as a low efficiency of drug delivery since a high percentage of the drug often remains in the device or deposits in the upper airways. Patients must be reasonably motivated, and often physically adept in manipulating and employing the delivery devices to ensure maximal efficiency. Drug delivery via the lungs requires a much higher degree of patient participation in the delivery process compared to the much more passive role required in swallowing a tablet or capsule. Co-ordination of drug delivery with the appropriate stage of inspiration or ensuring a sufficient air flow to actuate devices can be a problem for a number of patients. In addition, since corticosteroids are one of the major classes of drugs routinely administered via this route, associated side effects can include a degree of immune suppression and more frequently, oral candidiasis.

**Table 4.1. Advantages and disadvantages of dry powder inhalers.
Adapted from Ashurst, I. et al., Pharmaceutical
Science & Technology Today, 3(7), 246-256, 2000)**

Advantages	Disadvantages
• propellant-free • less need for patient coordination • less potential for formulation problems • less potential for extracting from the device component	• dependency on patient's inspiratory flow rate and profile • device resistance and other design issues • greater potential problem in dose uniformity • less protection from environmental effects and patient abuse • more expensive than pMDI • not available worldwide

DPIs are versatile delivery systems that may require some degree of dexterity to operate. Its formulation may consist of the drug alone or of drug blended with a carrier material which is usually lactose. The advantages and disadvantages of DPIs are summarized in Table 4.1. DPIs in common use today are breath actuated, and the energy for dry powder dispersion and generation of the aerosol are derived from the patient's inhalation. This method alleviates the problem of coordination of actuation and inhalation that many patients have with pMDIs, but several studies have shown that the dosing performance of some DPIs, in terms of total dose or fine particle dose emitted from the device, is dependent on the inspiratory flow rate. One of the key factors involved in optimizing DPI's performance is the precise particle engineering required to produce a powder formulation that delivers an accurate, consistent and efficient dose of the drug (Telko and Hickey 2005).

Dry powder formulations are activated and driven by the patients' inspiratory flow. Furthermore, the generation of aerosol often requires a high inspiratory flow rate to complete the emitted dose. DPIs may cause coughing. These devices are not recommended for children under the age of five, people with severe asthma or those suffering a severe attack. All DPIs have four basic features: a dose metering mechanism, an aerosolization mechanism, a deaggregation mechanism and an adapter to direct the aerosol into the patient's mouth.

4.2. Factors Affecting Dry Powder Inhaler Performance

From the physiology of the pulmonary system, drug deposition will be related to pulmonary physiology. In general, an appropriate particle size should be in the range of 0.5-5 µm. While using a fine particle of the drug, it will produce more surface free energy. Drug aerosol particles will attach firmly to surfaces they contact and form agglomerates by the cohesive force. This is called drug-drug aggregate formulation.

The drug-drug agglomerate formulations produce difficulties in generating the release of aerosol particle. Filled with an appropriate size of coarser carrier particle of about 35 µm the drug particles will form weak adhesive forces (Figure 4.1) that result in an improved percentage of fine drug particle by reducing the force needed to deagglomerate drug particle and improve a uniformity of the dosage form (Broadhead, Rouan, and Rhodes 1995). This is called the drug-carrier aggregates formulation. Sometimes fine particles of a tertiary component (e.g., leucine, lecithin or magnesium stearate) are used to adjust the interfacial properties of the carrier particles. They decrease the drug-carrier adhesion force and lead to producing a greater percent of the fine particle fraction (%FPF) of the drug (Begat et al. 2004).

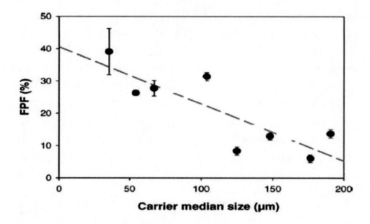

Figure 4.1. Relationship between the %FPF (mean ± S.D., n = 5) and the carrier median diameter. (Adapted from Louey, M. D. et al., *International Journal of Pharmaceutics,* 252(1-2), 87-98, 2003).

The important forces in the formulation are the cohesive and adhesive forces. To improve deposition to the deep lung, fine drug particles must be generated by reducing the cohesive force and forming a weak adhesive force (Figure 4.2). The small drug particles have a high surface cohesive force and form self-aggregates that are hard to deagglomerate. The method to produce weak adhesive forces between drug-carrier particles by adding adhering micronized carrier particles on the surface of the coarse lactose particle (Louey, Razia, and Stewart 2003). The carrier roughness can be reduced by surface treatment of the carrier particle and/or filled with other excipients.

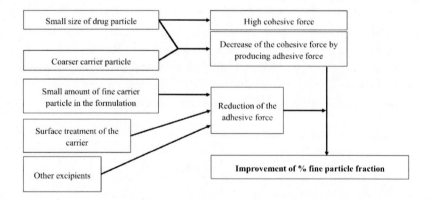

Figure 4.2. Methodology to reduce the cohesive force and forming a weak adhesive force.

DPIs can be developed by proper device design and powder technology. Two factors are important in powder technology; the cohesive forces and the flowability. Powder dispersibility is controlled by the interparticle cohesive forces which are proportional to the area of contact and separation distance between the particles (Weers and Miller 2015). Strong interparticle forces lead to a poor powder flow. The active drug substance needed in a DPI formulation is a micronized drug. The smaller the particles, the stronger the cohesive forces (Ahmad, Ungphaiboon, and Srichana (2015 and drug aggregates cause poor flowability. To improve flowability, there are two ways to prepare the formulations; with or without a carrier.

4.3. Formulations without Carrier

Only micronized drug particles form loose aggregates in the formulation. These loosely aggregated drug particles (spheroids) can be prepared by the controlled agglomeration of micronized particles. Spheroids have large particle sizes around 0.5 mm in diameter and thus have appropriate flow properties. Of course, spheroids exhibit better flow properties than micronized material. They carry low static charge during handling and operation (Healy et al. 2014). When spheroids are loaded into the DPI, they break up into primary particles during inhalation. It has been reported that the major disadvantage of such systems containing spheroids is the high variability in the emitted dose. Another technology to prepare spheres is to coat the particles with leucine (Pilcer and Amighi 2010, Raula, Lähde, and Kauppinen 2009).

Figure 4.3 shows the primary particles forming aggregates and agglomerates. The size of the primary particles increases as they form aggregates and when the aggregates bind together they form agglomerates.

4.4. Formulations with a Carrier

The majority of marketed drugs use carriers to improve flowability and reproducibility of dosing. Commonly used carriers are lactose and glucose. Other carriers that have been investigated are mannitol, sorbitol, maltitol, xylitol and arabinose (Steckel and Brandes 2004, Rahimpour, Kouhsoltani, and Hamishehkar 2014). Coarse carriers can increase the flowability which leads to an increase in the quantity of the drug reaching the lower airways. The dispersion properties depend on the performance of the drug aggregates on the carrier surface (Louey, Razia, and Stewart 2003). Aggregation not only requires much more appropriate forces for uniform drug dispersion but also an appropriate strength of the inspiration force to deaggregate the drug from the carrier. The drug aggregation patterns are of 4 types: drug aggregate on the carrier, fine drug particles, aggregate of fine drug particles and the aggregate of fine drug particle and carriers (Srichana, Martin, and Marriott 2000).

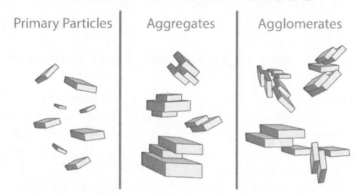

Figure 4.3. Features of primary particles, aggregates, and agglomerates.

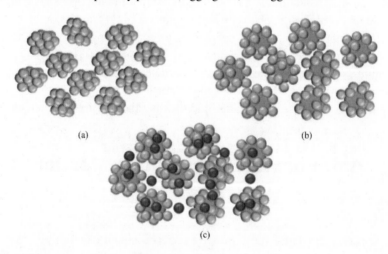

Figure 4.4. Interaction between particles drug-drug aggregates (a), drug-carrier aggregates (b), drug-carrier aggregates with "tertiary component" that are shown in small dark particles (c).

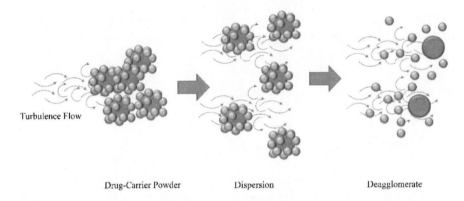

Turbulence Flow

Drug-Carrier Powder   Dispersion   Deagglomerate

Figure 4.5. Dispersion and deaggregation of the drug from the carrier by turbulent flow. Orange circle represents the carrier particles, green circle represents drug particles.

When the inspiratory flow is applied, the turbulent flow of the inspiration causes drug dispersion and deaggregation of the drug from the carrier (Figure 4.5). The drug will travel to the lower respiratory tract and alveoli while carriers which have a larger size are deposited on the oropharyngeal regions. Drug deposition in the lungs ranges from 15-40% of the emitted dose with current DPI devices (Anderson 2001).

In the development of the dry powder formulations, the following factors should be considered:

4.4.1. Particle Size of the Drug

Control of particle size may be used as a tool to target aerosol to the site of action. Particles larger than 10 μm will deposit on the oropharynx while particles smaller than 0.5 μm can be exhaled. Particle sizes larger than 5 μm may deposit on the bronchiolar regions, whereas the 1-3 μm particles can reach the alveoli (Gupta and Hickey 1991, Zanen, Go, and Lammers 1994). Therefore, the desirable size of an inhaled particle should be less than 5 μm and a suitable size for bronchodilator drug must be in the range of 0.5-5 μm. Most drug particles that have decreased sizes due to different processing technologies will be explained later in this chapter. Also, the drug particles can be categorized at least into organic and inorganic compounds that behave differently in terms of their size. Besides the chemical constituents of the molecule, the crystalline and amorphous states are also the important factors to be considered. From our experience working with salbutamol sulfate, budesonide, amphotericin B, rifampicin, isoniazid, pyrazinamide, ethambutol hydrochloride and levofloxacin, all of these molecules are very different in their class solubility that affects their physicochemical properties. In all cases, the size has to be carefully controlled.

4.4.2. Particle Size of the Carrier

A carrier is employed to improve the flowability of the fine drug particle. Therefore, it must be easy to handle and reproduce in the filling process. The incorporation of the carrier may cause irritation, coughing and bronchoconstriction (Timsina et al. 1994). Some studies have shown the effects of the particle size of a carrier on the efficiency of the formulation delivery. When the carrier size was decreased, the respirable fraction increased (Rahimpour and Hamishehkar 2012). However, the exploitation of this method was limited because of the aggregation of fine carrier particles (Ganderton 1999). The most suitable carrier size was approximately 30-90 µm.

When defining the particle size of the aerosols, it is also important to take into account the density, shape, surface roughness and geometric diameter, since all of these parameters affect the aerodynamic diameter of the inhaled airstream. In view of this, the MMAD can be useful in describing the diameter of the particles that differ in physical characteristics. Similar to the drug, the carriers can be grouped into different classes from the very water soluble sugar, cyclic sugar, phospholipids, amino acids, bile salts to polymer molecules (chitosan and PLGA) as detailed in Chapter 5. The carrier particle is also different and difficult to control and requires different comminution technology to obtain the appropriate size. All carriers behave differently in terms of their moisture sorption, crystallinity, electrostatic charges and all will influence the processing condition, handling, and storage.

Particle size is the predominant factor that governs the physical properties of the powder. The determination and control of the particle size are often an essential requirement in the formulation of pharmaceuticals. This is particularly true in the formulation of dry powders for inhalation, since the particle size of both the carrier and drug particles determines the powder performance at every stage that affects the flowability, fluidization, separation and deposition of powders. The importance of particle size in the development of solid pharmaceutical dosage forms has long been appreciated and techniques for its measurement are well established. However, the particle size obtained is dependent upon the principle of measurement (see Chapter 1).

4.4.3. Particle Shape

Particle shape is one of the most intractable and uncontrollable factors in powder technology. Different generation methods for the same material will almost always result in the production of particles of different particle shape. The packing patterns of anisometric particles, such as those with a high elongation or flatness ratio, are largely dependent on the processing conditions that the powder has experienced. Powder handling, such as mixing, compression, and vibration, may introduce enough energy to the powder such that its component particles tend to orientate themselves to the most stable conformations.

Particles having a more irregular shape exhibit much higher porosities in powder beds than spherical particles, both before and after tapping. Theoretically, irregular particles should exhibit higher adhesion forces than more spherical particles of a similar mass under the same conditions, if the microscopic factors are negligible and the particles seek the most stable orientation on the substrate surface. Particle shape may affect the flow properties of a powder by changing interparticulate and/or frictional forces between the particles. In general, if the particle shape can reduce both interparticulate and frictional forces, then it is said to be favorable for a good powder flow. The effect of the particle shape on the powder flow is more complicated than the particle size. Materials of different mechanical properties would need to possess a unique particle shape for optimized processing and this may change in different processing conditions.

4.4.4. Drug and Carrier Surface

Generally, dry powder aerosols are made by mixing the micronized drug and large carrier particle (Sawatdee 2005). The mechanical stability of these ordered powder mixtures is highly influenced by the surface properties of the carrier (Lai and Hersey 1987, Staniforth et al. 1982). Only limited areas show a high binding affinity. Redispersion of the drug from the carrier surface during inhalation is the most critical factor. Control of the crystallization conditions to produce a smooth carrier surface has been reported to restrict adhesion and enhance separation (Ganderton 1999, Zeng et al. 2000, Park, Park, and Choi 2014).

A carrier surface has a surface porosity. Pore size on the carrier surface can be characterized into 3 size groups that are nanopores (0.007-1.00 µm), micropores (1.00-8.06 µm) and macropores (8.06-150 µm) (Ahuja and Pathak 2009, Fan, Zhang, and Wang 2013). Nanopores reduce the effective carrier contact area and increase the distance between drug and carrier particles. Nanopores thus reduce the magnitude of interparticulate adhesion forces in an inhalation mixture. Microporosity carriers do not play important roles during the aerosolization process. They contribute to the mixing process by increasing the effectiveness of the cohesive drug agglomerates, de-agglomeration and distribution of drug particles over the carrier surface. On the other hand, macroporous carriers apparently have a negative influence on the performance. When the grooves are introduced on carrier they will prevent drug particles from the drag and lift from the carrier surface (Shalash, Molokhia, and Elsayed 2015).

Carrier surface coating is an effective technique to improve the carrier surface characteristics. Lactose carrier particles that were coated with a thin layer of magnesium stearate by physical mixing enhanced the *in vitro* inhalation performance of the formulation when compared to the uncoated lactose formulations (Iida et al. 2004). Coating leucine or magnesium stearate on drug particles is also reported (Raula et al. 2012, Zhou et al. 2013). The particle morphology and surface roughness can be modified by spraying with bovine serum albumin to create either wrinkled or corrugated particles (Adi et al. 2008).

4.4.5 Drug Carrier Ratio

The respirable fraction increased when the drug carrier ratio increased (Kassem 1990). This was due to the increase in the active binding sites as a higher drug concentration was able to bind to the lower affinity sites or be free. Recent studies had revealed that when the drug to carrier surface coverage was more than a monolayer, the aerosol performance was decreased (Young et al. 2011, Grasmeijer et al. 2013). Although there are wide ranges of drug contents in various formulations, it has been a common practice to use a fixed drug to carrier ratio of 1:67.5 in the studies. This ratio was most likely adopted from earlier carrier based formulations for the Rotahaler®, Diskhaler® and Cyclohaler®. It is well known that drug content affects the homogeneity blend and the drug detachment from the carrier. Adhesive mixtures are a dynamic process of ordering and randomization that determines the outcome of the blending process. With increased drug content, the equilibrium is displaced towards randomization which results in a less homogeneous mixture that is more prone to segregation during handling. This adverse effect may produce a better drug detachment from the carrier particles when the separation forces are generated. Several mechanisms have been postulated to explain the effect of the drug content on the dispersion performance of adhesive mixtures for inhalation. First, the so-called active sites on the lactose carrier surface may become saturated with increased drug content. This results in a decrease in the mass of the drug that adheres strongly to the carrier surface and improves the detachment of the drug particle. Second, the formation of a layer or an agglomeration of the drug particles with an increase in the drug content can cause detachment of the large agglomerates rather than the single drug particles, if a failure in adhesive bond formation between the inner drug layer and the carrier surface occurs during inhalation. This too may improve drug detachment, because it increases the magnitude of the lift and inertial separation forces to become more than that of the interaction forces of the drug carrier. Third, a higher drug content increases, drug particles will fill up the clefts and depressions in the carrier surface. By being transferred through the powder bed, this enables to act effectively as press-on forces on the drug particles that would have found shelter from them in carrier surface irregularities at a much lower drug content. It causes the particle interaction forces to increase by reducing their separation distance and increasing their contact surface area, and therefore, it causes drug detachment to be negatively affected. Lastly, it was hypothesized that with increased drug content, detached particles might be more likely to collide with neighboring drug particles to cause an enhanced drug detachment which is a mechanism referred to as the 'collision effect' (Grasmeijer et al. 2013). Collision effects may marginally contribute to improve drug detachment with an increase in the drug content.

4.4.6 The Use of Tertiary Component and Mixing Sequence

The addition of the tertiary components affects the deaggregation and deposition of aerosols. The addition of magnesium stearate reduced the adhesion between drug and carrier, leading to the loss of homogeneity and destabilization (Staniforth et al. 1982, Lai and Hersey 1987, Kassem 1990,

Zeng et al. 1999). When the magnesium stearate concentration was increased, the adhesion between the drug and carrier decreased and resulted in an increase in the respirable fraction. Furthermore, different mixing sequences were shown to result in different deposition profiles (Zeng et al. 1999). High-energy active sites may exist on the coarse carriers for the drug to preferentially adhere due to stronger interactions (Ahmad, Ungphaiboon, and Srichana 2015). When fine carriers of a tertiary component are added, they will compete with the drugs for the active sites, making the drug easier to detach from the carrier during inhalation. Based on this observation, the active sites can be saturated. Thus the sequence of mixing the drug, coarse carrier and tertiary component is expected to be critical. Furthermore, high-energy sites on the carrier surface were still observed after the addition of the tertiary component (Chan 2006). A proposed mechanism that may involve the formation of weak conglomerates between the drug, carrier and tertiary component was developed. In this case, the drug distribution between the coarse carrier and tertiary component may cause a disruption of attractive interactions in the conglomerate.

4.5. Electrostatic Charge

Electrostatic charges also play important roles in dry powder aerosols (Finlay 2001). Although human studies are limited, an *in silico* study has shown that for aerosols with 200 charges per particle, electrostatic forces become predominant (Balachandran et al. 1997). Byron et al. (1997) found that a fine particle dose charge that ranged from -400 pC to 200 pC for Bricanyl® and Pulmicort®. Kwok et al. (2011) also reported the effect of the relative humidity on the electrostatic charge of DPI using an electrical low-pressure impactor. Both Bricanyl® and Pulmicort® displayed a different charge distribution and a bipolar charge across 0.388 µm to 6.06 µm. The effect of the relative humidity on charging the dry powder aerosol appeared to be dependent on the drug. A comprehensive review on the role of electrostatic charge in pharmaceutical aerosol was performed by Wong, Chan, and Kwok (2013) and Kaialy (2016).

4.6. Particle Production Technology

Comminution technology has been introduced into aerosol science to prepare powder particles. Milling, high-pressure homogenization, spray drying, spray freeze- drying, crystallization, supercritical fluid and adsorption/coacervation technology have been used in aerosol science. However, the particle size is not well established during these processes. The size of the drug particles must be reduced to the respirable size range in a separate unit operation. There are many options and it may be necessary to find the one that works best for any specific drug. In the dry powder aerosols production, several techniques are employed to decrease the particle to an appropriate size (Table 4.2).

**Table 4.2. Techniques commonly used in particle
production for dry powder inhalers**

Technique	Comments	References
Jet milling/Wet milling	Commercially established for numerous inhalation drugs. No subsequent separation process required. Introducing an amorphous content. Generally, difficult to scale up. Concerns with respect to foreign particulate material from the erosion of the milling media.	Irngartinger et al. (2004) Telko and Hickey (2005) Rasenack (2010) Nakpheng et al. (2011) Jetmalani et al. (2012)
High-pressure Homogenization	Commercially used for several inhalation drugs. Nanosuspension particle. Liposome formulation.	Rabinow (2004) Chougule, Padhi, and Misra (2007) Xu, Mansour, and Hickey (2011)
Spray drying	Commercially proved Single-step particle formation process. Control over size, morphology, density and surface composition. Process development required to minimize process-induced degradation.	White et al. (2005) Chen et al. (2005) White et al. (2005) Chow et al. (2007) Vehring (2008)

Technique	Comments	References
Spray freeze-drying	Two-step process (freezing and lyophilization). Very low-density, fragile particles. Energy-intensive, complex process. Freezing stress, but no thermal degradation.	Leuenberger (2002) Rogers, Johnston, and Williams (2003) Wang et al. (2012) Ali and Lamprecht (2014)
Controlled crystallization	More stable product. Control physical form of active ingredients, polymorphic forms formation.	Beach et al. (1999) Havelund (2001) Rasenack, Steckel, and Muller (2003)
	Particle engineering of inhaled drugs.	Rasenack and Muller (2004) Steckel, Rasenack, and Muller (2003) Ikegami et al. (2000), (2002) Voss and Finlay (2002)
Supercritical fluid RESS Supercritical fluid SAS	Limited drugs soluble in the supercritical fluid. Drug must be poorly soluble in the supercritical fluid.	Steckel, Thies, and Müller (1997) Steckel and Muller (1998) Velaga, Berger, and Carlfors (2002) Shekunov et al. (2003) Rehman et al. (2004)
Adsorption/ coacervation	Complex/several critical parameters.	Alvim and Grosso (2010) Yadidi (2016)

4.6.1. Comminution by Jet Milling/Wet Mill

The common comminution technique is milling. There are three types of mills that are able to reduce the particle size to 2–5 μm. These are jet mill; pin-mill and ball mill.

Mechanical processing, such as milling has been shown to affect the crystallinity of the material; this effect must be considered. Jet milling (or air attrition milling) is the most useful technique; it reduces the particle size via high-velocity particle–particle collisions. Unmilled particles are introduced into the milling chamber. High-pressure nitrogen is fed through nozzles and accelerates the solid particles to sonic velocities. The particles collide and fracture. While flying around the mill, larger particles are subjected to a higher centrifugal force and are forced to the outer perimeter of the chamber (Figure 4.6). Small particles exit the mill through the central discharge stream. Depending on the nitrogen pressure and powder feed rate, particles down to 1 μm in diameter can be produced.

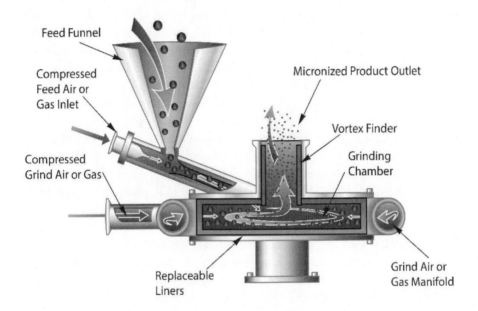

Figure 4.6. Air jet mill (Adapted from www.umamicron.com).

A pin mill uses a mechanical impact to grind material, both by particle–particle and particle-solid collisions. A pin mill is equipped with a series of concentrically mounted pins located on a spinning rotor and a stationary stator plate. The powder is fed to the milling chamber and transported through the milling chamber by centrifugal force. The milled product is collected from the bottom. The pin mill can produce 1 μm particles, but not as small as the jet mill. On the other hand, the power consumption of a pin mill is lower than that of the jet mill.

The ball mill is essentially a rotating cylinder loaded with the drug and "milling media" (i.e., balls that grind the drug between each other as they tumble inside the mill). The size and material of the milling media can be varied. Ball milling is very slow and the process is poorly scalable, which is why tumbling ball mills are used only in the laboratory.

DPI inhalation products contain the micronized drug in either an agglomerate or blend. Such particles are normally produced by crystallization, followed by filtering, drying and micronization (Jetmalani et al. 2012). The particle size can be reduced by attrition, impaction or shear force. Air jet-milling is well-established to manufacture dry powders for inhalation. Although milling can be performed on a dry or wet basis, dry grinding is more commonly employed as it is less labor-intensive. In the jet milling process, the starting material undergoes many impact events until a quantity of the required particle size fraction is achieved and separated from the larger particles by inertial impaction. This will ensure that the particle size required for respiratory delivery is eventually obtained. The obtained particle shape is either tabular or rounded. However, this milling process can be time-consuming and inefficient for organic pharmaceuticals and can adversely alter the surface and solid-state properties of the materials.

Micronization also generates electrostatic charges and amorphous domains on the particle surface. This will change the ground material to have both cohesive and adhesive properties. In some cases, the whole material bulk may become amorphous. As the amorphous domains are thermodynamically unstable, such amorphous products will recrystallize leading to crystal growth on the milled particle surface and formation of solid bridges between the particles. The material is also prone to chemical decomposition and water sorption. All of these physical and chemical changes are highly undesirable and can adversely affect the *in vitro* performance of the DPI formulations. The operating condition must be clearly defined such as temperatures and relative humidities. Since micronization may reduce drug stability, modified techniques are necessary to solve the problems of thermolabile biopharmaceuticals (Nakpheng et al. 2011). For example, micronization of the decapeptide cetrorelix can be done by suspending the drug in a fluid propellant coupled with a cryostat down to -70 °C, followed by evaporation of the fluid propellant to recover the micronized material (Irngartinger et al. 2004). This milling technique was effective and mild for the peptide, and perhaps better than spray drying because of the higher respirable fraction of the milled material.

4.6.2. High-Pressure Homogenization

High-pressure homogenization offers more advantages over traditional micronization. This technique can produce nanoparticles in sizes between 100 and 700 nm which can afford higher bioavailability and likely to obtain greater efficient drug delivery and rapid dissolution in the lung. The homogeneity of nanosuspensions is also superior over the microparticulate suspensions and leads to a higher delivered dose with better dose uniformity (Figure 4.7) (Rabinow 2004).

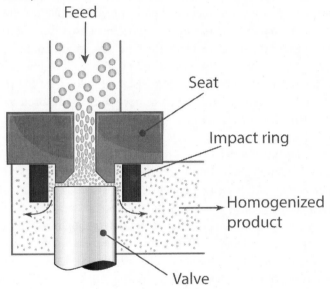

Figure 4.7. High-pressure homogenization (Adapted from https://en.wikipedia.org).

Typically, 20-30% w/w of the surfactant is required to stabilize the nanosuspensions. This amount is directly proportional to the specific surface area. The potential problems of this technique are from potential contamination with the grinding media and adverse effects of the high temperature on the chemical stability. These problems may be minimized or overcome by utilizing direct nanoparticle precipitation.

4.6.3. Spray Drying

Spray drying (SD) technology is very popular in the processing of food, biochemicals, and pharmaceutical materials. The technology is easy to operate, available to large scale-up, and able to produce composite materials. This technique can produce particle sizes in the range of 1-5 μm. The physical instability and thermal degradation of the products is a major concern of this method. This approach is rapidly expanding in a range of applications as the technology becomes more advanced. A typical SD process consists of four steps (Chow et al. 2007): (a) atomization of the feed solution; (b) sprayed droplets contact with hot gas; (c) drying of sprayed droplets and (d) separation of dried product (Figure 4.8). For each operating step, a variety of process designs varies depending on specific applications. The atomization can be generated from rotary atomizers, pressure nozzle or two fluid nozzles while air/fluid flow inside; the drying chamber can be co-current, counter-current or a mixed flow type. More recently, four-fluid nozzles with in-line mixing have been developed for the production of composite particles. The SD process can also be operated in different modes such as open cycle and closed cycle, semi-closed cycle with or without aseptic controls. The system can be further modified on a larger production scale and for better product recovery. For example, the bag-filter is replaced with a cyclone system or the product is dried at a lower inlet air temperature for thermolabile materials. The design of a high-efficiency cyclone separation system is also essential for industrial scale production.

The spray drying technique can be optimized to obtain suitable conditions for a particular product. Both product concentration and atomization rate can be manipulated to produce particles with different surface corrugations. In some cases, proper humidity control of the drying gas can afford particles with the desirable densities or aerodynamic diameters for pulmonary delivery (Chen et al. 2005).

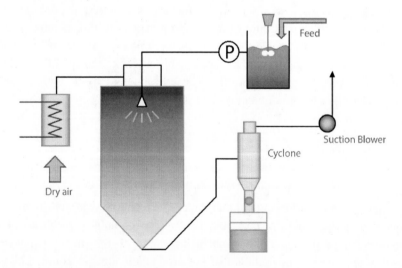

Figure 4.8. Spray drying (Adapted from www.eurotherm.com).

4.6.4. Spray Freeze-Drying

A typical spray freeze-drying (SFD) technique involves the atomization of an aqueous solution of a drug via an ultrasonic nozzle into a spray chamber filled with cryogenic liquid nitrogen. The spraying process can be performed above the surface of the cryogenic liquid or in the liquid depending on the position of the nozzle (Figure 4.9). Since the cryogenic liquid will decrease due to evaporation, continuous addition of fresh cryogenic liquid is required, especially when a longer atomization process or a large spray volume is used. The droplets solidify rapidly upon contact with the cryogenic liquid because of the high heat-transfer rate. Stirring of the cryogenic liquid may be required to prevent the possible aggregation of frozen particles. Once the spraying process is completed, the whole content can be freeze dried as with conventional freeze-drying. The sublimation of the spray solvent has also been developed (Leuenberger 2002, Rogers, Johnston, and Williams 2003). This process involves drying of the frozen particles by a stream of cold dry air inside an insulated stainless steel vessel. Changes of the moisture content in the product can be monitored, without interrupting the drying process.

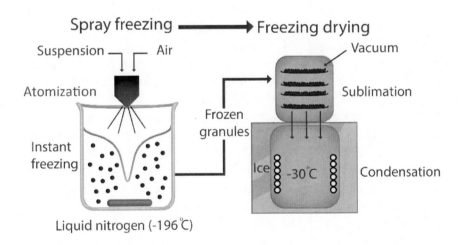

Figure 4.9. Spray freeze-drying (Adapted from http://powderpro.se).

Spray freeze-dried particles can be engineered to the desired particle size below 5 μm. The most important operating parameter is the mass ratio of the liquid feed to the atomized nitrogen. A decrease in the particle size can be achieved by a decrease in the mass ratio, while the addition of excipients may lead to an increase in the particle size. Further, the spray-freezing process has been modified; the drug solution is atomized and frozen simultaneously by mixing with a liquefied gas or supercritical fluid, such as supercritical CO_2. The liquid droplets are first dispersed with a static mixer within the supercritical CO_2 and then frozen. After spray freezing, the frozen solvent is removed, as in the case of freezing with cryogenic liquids, by vacuum or atmospheric freeze-drying. The large surface area and loose porous structure of the powder allow relatively fast drying compared to a standard lyophilization process.

4.6.5. Controlled Crystallization

Crystallization of hydrophobic drugs can be obtained by antisolvent precipitation (Rasenack, Steckel, and Muller 2003, Rasenack and Muller 2004). The precipitated crystals (e.g., budesonide, prednisolone, fluticasone and disodium cromoglycate) have been shown to exhibit a higher FPF than the jet-milled samples (Rasenack, Steckel, and Muller 2003, Steckel, Rasenack, and Muller 2003). Also, higher drug concentrations yield smaller particles. The amorphous content of such drugs is lower than that of the micronized samples, thus better physical stability can be obtained. Zinc-free insulin crystals have been prepared in a size range of 0.2-5 µm. The precipitated insulin crystals were more stable than those powders prepared by spray-drying, freeze-drying or oven drying (Havelund 2001).

Direct crystallization of spherical agglomerates has been utilized in pulmonary delivery formulations. This technique involves antisolvent precipitation of a drug solution in an organic solvent, followed by addition of water or a partially miscible organic solvent with water. For example, the introduction of ethyl acetate into the water/acetone crystallization medium resulted in the formation of spherical agglomerates (200-300 µm). Primary crystals were in the respirable range (d_{50} = 1.3-2.7 µm) (Ikegami et al. 2002, Ikegami et al. 2000). The agglomerated crystals deaggregate into primary particles upon mixing with lactose carrier. The adhered primary crystals were easily detached from the lactose during inhalation (Voss and Finlay 2002). Spherical crystallization can be achieved for certain drugs by quenching of a hot organic or aqueous drug solution with a cold organic or aqueous organic solvent. The quench solvent should be miscible with the drug solution. For instance, spherical microcrystals of salmeterol xinafoate, a long-acting antiasthmatic agent, can be readily produced by adding a hot propanol containing the drug to a chilled quench solvent (Beach et al. 1999). The agglomerates are free-flowing and readily micronizable to a suitable inhalable material.

The particle size control in all crystallization is the most challenging task because most molecules tend to form large crystals. The nucleation and growth mechanisms yield particles in the size range of 10-100 μm. Mixing between the drug solution and non-solvent can be fast agitation, high-velocity mixing or ultrasonic mixing. In the ultrasonic crystallization, the particle size can be controlled by the sonic-induced mixing and cavitation on supersaturation and nucleation. This mechanism renders more uniform particles. The mean particle size decreases if high concentrations of growth-retarding excipients are employed.

These growth retardants are compound-specific in terms of their interaction with the crystal surfaces. Furthermore, the use of additives designed to inhibit crystal growth is very strict due to purity control and toxicity issues. Finally, crystalline particles with a narrow size distribution are feasible with controlled crystallization. A major drawback of such a process is the need to remove all additives completely. The latter processing steps are not straightforward. This step may result in powder caking, impure samples and low dispersible powder.

4.6.6. Supercritical Fluid

A supercritical fluid (SCF) is a compressible liquid having gas transport properties. SCF exhibits pressure-tunable solubility, which is suitable for recrystallization operations. The most common SCF uses liquid carbon dioxide (CO_2) as a solvent. The SCF technique can be categorized into rapid expansion of supercritical solutions (RESS) and antisolvents (SAS). Schiavone et al. (2004) noted that a product prepared by SCFs yielded smoother budesonide particles, with less surface area than a milled drug. Particle engineering with SCFs is the subject of intensive research in the pharmaceutical industry; excellent reviews on this topic have been published elsewhere (Telko and Hickey 2005, Tabernero, Martín del Valle, and Galán 2012).

SCFs possess several advantages as solvents (or antisolvents) for pharmaceutical manufacturing. Supercritical CO_2 (SC-CO_2) is the most common SCF because of its low critical temperature (31.1°C), moderate pressure (73.8 bars), non-toxic inert nature and low cost. Despite the fact that SCF technology is often associated with SAS, several existing technologies differ in the applicability of the material. One of the most important physical attributes of the SC-CO$_2$ processing is the efficient extraction process. This often enables the production in a dry form or as an aqueous suspension. It promotes a clean and recycled precipitation process at low temperatures. The SCFs can be utilized for plasticization of polymers. SCFs have been used for the direct production of pure and composite particles with the advantages of selective precipitation and control of the crystalline forms. In SC-CO$_2$ applications, such as particle engineering of high potency and sensitive drugs, SC-CO$_2$ can reduce manufacturing complexity, energy, and solvent requirements.

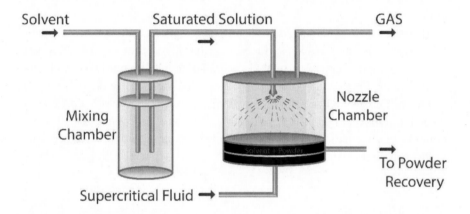

Figure 4.10. Supercritical fluid antisolvent systems (Adapted from http://eng.ege.edu.tr).

In all SAS processes, the mechanism is based on the rapid precipitation when a drug solution comes in contact with a SC-CO$_2$ (Figure 4.10). It is important to note that the mechanism of SAS changes under different pressures and temperature conditions. It depends on the solvent composition, known as the mixtures critical point. In the higher pressure, lower temperature phase region, the solvents are completely miscible, and the SAS proceeds as a typical precipitation process. In the lower pressure, higher temperature region, however, the SAS shifts towards a spraying extraction. Different SAS modifications are distinguished by mixing between the solution and SC-CO$_2$ feeds. For example, solution enhanced dispersion with SCF utilizes high-velocity mixing in a multi-component nozzle. Most of the drugs have very limited solubility in CO$_2$, SAS processes have attracted much attention in recent years because they offer a method for production of micronized dry powders. Most of the studies to date have focused on small molecules for inhalation.

For example, production of steroids has been demonstrated including budesonide and fluticasone (Steckel and Muller 1998, Steckel, Thies, and Müller 1997). Coated particles produced with SAS showed a significant increase in FPF when compared to the jet-milled products. It has been shown that SAS-produced powders exhibit non-spherical particles with a lower bulk density than micronized materials. Although the SC-CO_2 process produces particles with larger aerodynamic diameters than the micronized materials, they have a significantly higher FPF. An analysis of hydrocortisone particles using a multistage liquid impinger showed that the delivered dose increased by 30-40% for the SAS processed materials relative to the micronized particles (Velaga, Berger, and Carlfors 2002). The improved properties of the SAS-processed particles can be explained by the weak surface adhesion of these particles to the inhaler reservoir. The size reduction process in SAS needs to be optimized to obtain particles in the respirable range with the required shape. For such optimization, nozzles may suffer from the inefficient macro-mixing and periodic blockage, both of which can result in a broadening of the PSD. To address some of these problems, an SCF technology utilizing a turbulent-shear mixing system has been developed (Shekunov et al. 2003).

SAS processes possess a very important advantage to control the physical form of the drug. Controlled production of different polymorphic forms has been demonstrated by varying the working conditions. The produced materials are usually crystalline and have a low residual solvent content. Engineering of the hydrates, solvates and amorphous solids by SAS processing has also been reported (Steckel, Thies, and Müller 1997, Steckel and Muller 1998, Velaga, Berger, and Carlfors 2002, Rehman et al. 2004, Shekunov et al. 2003).

4.6.7. Adsorption/Coacervation Particle Formation

Adsorption was employed to produce sodium cromoglycate adsorbed with fatty acids (Fults, Miller, and Hickey 1997). The coated lauric and stearic acids led to an increase in the FPFs. The lauric acid appeared to alter the deposition by changing the particle to a more elongated shape compared to the untreated sample. Whereas, the stearic acid had an altered particle shape to a smaller degree but had better FPFs due to the reduced interparticulate interactions.

Coacervation is a phase separation phenomenon that occurs in a solution of two liquid phases containing a solute species with polymer-rich and solvent-rich phases. The process is reported to be scalable, although it requires a multi-step particle separation: (A) a homogeneous polymer solution, (B) phase separation and coacervation droplets, (C) deposition of coating and (D) membrane formation. The physical chemistry of any coacervation process is complex and has several critical parameters. It usually involves large molecular weight polymers. Coacervation can be controlled by temperature change, solution composition and pH. A more complex coacervation may involve deposition of a shell material around the encapsulated core drug (Figure 4.11). Coacervation followed by hardening of the dispersed phase generates solid particles. This technique has been employed in DPI to produce insulin and α-1-antitrypsin. The technology used a temperature controlled coacervation in the presence of polyethylene glycol (PEG). Subsequent dialysis was carried out against an aqueous solution followed by centrifugation to remove the PEG and then lyophilization. Both drugs were solid spheres with MMADs of 2.7-2.9 μm. This process gained advantages from the utilization of an aqueous system that was suitable for the production of protein spheres. Further investigation into its applicability to small molecules and protein formulations is certainly worthwhile and will be challenging.

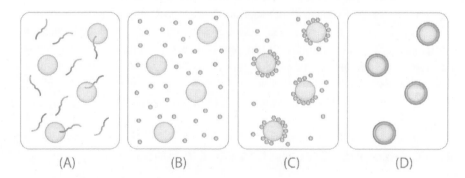

(A)   (B)   (C)   (D)

Figure 4.11. Coacervation process.

4.7. Processing Conditions

The mixing time for each drug and carrier should be optimized because an extension of the mixing time increased the drug particle association to the active surface of the carrier, and consequently, increased the stability and decreased the dispersibility (Ganderton 1999). The processes involved in a powder formulation have been extensively reviewed in the pharmaceutical technology/engineering area. After the drug and excipient(s) have individually been brought to their desired forms, they are combined in the blending process (Saleem, Smyth, and Telko 2008). The importance of the blending process can be easily overlooked. However, it is a critical step for the manufacture of a DPI product and is in fact subjected to substantial optimization work during development.

When mixing powders with different properties, particle sizes and ratios, as is the case with DPI formulations, inadequate mixing can cause poor dose uniformity. In many cases, inadequate mixing cannot be overcome simply by increasing the mixing time. Mixer selection, rotation speed, capacity and fill level are all subjected to optimization as they can all affect the blend homogeneity. Blending conditions also affect the interparticle forces which are a primary determinant by the FPF. Different powders may have different mixing requirements depending on the forces present between the various particles. For low concentration (drug-carrier ratio) blends, geometric dilutions are necessary preblending steps. The flow properties of the components of the powder blend will play an important role in the efficiency of blending and ultimately in an aerosol dispersion. Powder flow properties have been studied for some time and methods have been adopted for their characterization including bulk and tapped density, and the angle of repose.

Powder sampling is an important prerequisite for accurate characterization. Blending validation is an important activity required by good manufacturing practices in the United States Code of Federal Regulations. However, taking blend samples at different times to determine the uniformity of the blend is associated with several difficulties. New techniques are emerging that can determine the blend homogeneity without removal of samples from the mixer; techniques such as near-infrared and Fourier transform-infrared analysis can determine blend uniformity by the nondestructive acquisition of infrared spectra. After the formulation has been blended, it is filled into capsules, multi-dose blisters or reservoirs for use with the inhaler device. The filling process is automated and depends on the nature of the metering system.

4.8. Storage Conditions

Adhesion and dispersion of aerosols determine the efficacy of the formulation. Several parameters are involved in adhesion and dispersion such as rugosity, shape, surface, charge and moisture. Moisture content is the main factor that influences the cohesiveness of powder. An increase in cohesiveness with the rising moisture content is due to the adsorbed water. Hygroscopic aerosol particles will grow in size until the vapor pressure exerted by the droplet equals the vapor pressure of the water in the lung. The aerosols increase in size at high humidity as compared to low humidity (Hiller (1991. Hygroscopicity is the intrinsic tendency of material to take on moisture from its surroundings. Hygroscopicity is affected by the crystallinity of the material and the morphology of the particles. Hygroscopic drugs present a greater risk of physical and chemical instability. Moisture uptake and loss due to changes in relative humidity can result in local dissolution and recrystallization and lead to irreversible aggregation through solid bridge formation which can adversely affect the aerosol generation and lung deposition. Hygroscopicity can also alter the adhesive and cohesive properties or, in more extreme situations, substantially increase the particle size. Hygroscopic growth involves the uptake of moisture which will reach equilibrium in the droplets as a function of the water activity of the solutions formed and the surrounding atmosphere of water vapor. Hygroscopic growth has implications for the equilibrium moisture content of the particles in the dosage form prior to generation of the aerosol; it can cause chemical or physical instability of the product. For aerosols, the physical instability is more important, because agglomeration may be irreversible and lead to an inability to generate aerosol particles of respirable size. As aerosol particles enter the lungs, they experience an environment of high humidity (99.5% relative humidity at 37°C). Although they may not reach equilibrium during transit, susceptible aerosol particles may be subjected to hygroscopic growth that increases particle dimensions and affects lung deposition. Hygroscopic growth can be prevented by coating the drug particles with hydrophobic films. However, no such approach has been successfully implemented in a marketed formulation.

The equilibrium moisture content of a drug and excipient must be determined over a range of relative humidities so that storage conditions can be defined and other protective measures can also be considered. Excipients that modify the hygroscopic properties of a drug may need to be considered.

References

Adi, Santoso S., Handoko Adi, Patricia Tang, Daniela Traini, Hak-Kim Chan, and Paul M Young. 2008. "Micro-particle corrugation, adhesion and inhalation aerosol efficiency." *European Journal of Pharmaceutical Sciences* 35 (1-2):12-18. doi: 10.1016/j.ejps.2008.05.009.

Ahmad, Md Iftekhar, Suwipa Ungphaiboon, and Teerapol Srichana. 2015. "The development of dimple-shaped chitosan carrier for ethambutol dihydrochloride dry powder inhaler." *Drug Development and Industrial Pharmacy* 41 (5):791-800. doi: 10.3109/03639045.2014.903493.

Ahuja, Gaurav, and Kamla Pathak. 2009. "Porous carriers for controlled/modulated drug delivery." *Indian Journal of Pharmaceutical Sciences* 71 (6):599-607. doi: 10.4103/0250-474x.59540.

Ali, Mohamed Ehab Hab, and Alf Lamprecht. 2014. "Spray freeze drying for dry powder inhalation of nanoparticles." *European Journal of Pharmaceutics and Biopharmaceutics* 87 (3):510-7. doi: 10.1016/j.ejpb.2014.03.009.

Alvim, Izabela Dutra, and Carlos Raimundo Ferreira Grosso. 2010. "Microparticles obtained by complex coacervation: influence of the type of reticulation and the drying process on the release of the core material." *Food Science and Technology* 30:1069-1076.

Anderson, Paula J. 2001. "DElivery options and devices for aerosolized therapeutics*." *Chest* 120 (3_suppl):89S-93S. doi: 10.1378/chest.120.3_suppl.89S.

Ashurst, Ian, Ann Malton, David Prime, and Barry Sumby. 2000. "Latest advances in the development of dry powder inhalers." *Pharmaceutical Science & Technology Today* 3 (7):246-256. doi: 10.1016/S1461-5347(00)00275-3.

Balachandran, Wamadeva, Wojciech W. Machowski, E Gaura, and Chris J. Hudson. 1997. "Control of drug aerosol in human airways using electrostatic forces." *Journal of Electrostatics* 40:579-584.

Beach, Steve, David Latham, Colin Sidgwick, Mazen Hanna, and Peter York. 1999. "Control of the physical form of salmeterol xinafoate." *Organic Process Research & Development* 3 (5):370-376. doi: 10.1021/op990160z.

Begat, Philippe, David A. V. Morton, John N. Staniforth, and Robert Price. 2004. "The cohesive-adhesive balances in dry powder inhaler formulations II: Influence on fine particle delivery characteristics." *Pharmaceutical Research* 21 (10):1826-1834.

Broadhead, Joanne, Edmond S. K. Rouan, and Christopher T. Rhodes. 1995. "Dry-powder inhalers: evaluation of testing methodology and effect of inhaler design." *Pharmaceutica Acta Helvetiae* 70 (2):125-31.

Byron, Peter R., Joanne Peart, and John N. Staniforth. 1997. "Aerosol electrostatics. I: Properties of fine powders before and after aerosolization by dry powder inhalers." *Pharmaceutical Research* 14 (6):698-705.

Chan, Hak-Kim. 2006. "Dry powder aerosol drug delivery-Opportunities for colloid and surface scientists." *Colloids and Surfaces A: Physicochemical and Engineering Aspects* 284-285:50-55. doi: 10.1016/j.colsurfa. 2005.10.091.

Chen, Donghao, Richard P. Batycky, Lloyd Johnston, and Jeffrey Mintzes. 2005. Control of process humidity to produce large, porous particles. US Patents.

Chougule, Mahavir, Bijay Padhi, and Ambikanandan Misra. 2007. "Nano-liposomal dry powder inhaler of tacrolimus: Preparation, characterization, and pulmonary pharmacokinetics." *International Journal of Nanomedicine* 2 (4):675-688.

Chow, Albert, Henry Tong, Pratibhash Chattopadhyay, and Boris Shekunov. 2007. "Particle Engineering for Pulmonary Drug Delivery." *Pharmaceutical Research* 24 (3):411-437. doi: 10.1007/s11095-006-9174-3.

Fan, Ling, Junping Zhang, and Aiqin Wang. 2013. "In situ generation of sodium alginate/hydroxyapatite/halloysite nanotubes nanocomposite hydrogel beads as drug-controlled release matrices." *Journal of Materials Chemistry B* 1 (45):6261-6270. doi: 10.1039/c3tb20971g.

Finlay, Warren H. 2001. "1 - Introduction." In *The Mechanics of Inhaled Pharmaceutical Aerosols*, 1-2. London: Academic Press.

Fults, Kristen A., Irving F. Miller, and Anthony J Hickey. 1997. "Effect of particle morphology on emitted dose of fatty acid treated disodium cromoglycate powder aerosols." *Pharmaceutical Development and Technology* 2 (1):67-79. doi: 10.3109/10837459709022610.

Ganderton, David. 1999. "Pulmonary delivery: A testing decade." *Pharmaceutical Technology Europe* 11 (10):52.

Grasmeijer, Floris, Paul Hagedoorn, Henderik W. Frijlink, and Anne H. de Boer. 2013. "Drug content effects on the dispersion performance of adhesive mixtures for inhalation." *PLoS ONE* 8 (8):e71339. doi: 10.1371/journal.pone.0071339.

Gupta, Pramod K., and Anthony J. Hickey. 1991. "Contemporary approaches in aerosolized drug delivery to the lung." *Journal of Controlled Release* 17 (2):127-147. doi: 10.1016/0168-3659(91)90053-G.

Havelund, Svend. 2001. Pulmonary insulin crystals. Google Patents.

Healy, Anne Marie, Maria Ines Nes Amaro, Krzystof Jan An Paluch, and Lidia Tajber. 2014. "Dry powders for oral inhalation free of lactose carrier particles." *Advanced Drug Delivery Reviews* 75:32-52. doi: 10.1016/j.addr.2014.04.005.

Hiller, F. Charles. 1991. "Health Implications of Hygroscopic Particle Growth in the Human Respiratory Tract." *Journal of Aerosol Medicine* 4 (1):1-23. doi: 10.1089/jam.1991.4.1.

Iida, Kotaro, Yukari Inagaki, Hiroaki Todo, Hirokazu Okamoto, Kazumi Danjo, and Hans Luenberger. 2004. "Effects of surface processing of lactose carrier particles on dry powder inhalation properties of salbutamol sulfate." *Chemical & Pharmaceutical Bulletin* 52 (8):938-42.

Ikegami, Kazuhiko, Yoshiaki Kawashima, Hirofumi Takeuchi, Hiromitsu Yamamoto, Nobuyuki Isshiki, Den-ichi Momose, and Kiyohisa Ouchi. 2002. "Improved inhalation behavior of steroid KSR-592 in vitro with Jethaler by polymorphic transformation to needle-like crystals (beta-form)." *Pharmaceutical Research* 19 (10):1439-45.

Ikegami, Kazuhiko, Yoshiaki Kawashima, Hirofumi Takeuchi, Hiromitsu Yamamoto, Den-ichi Momose, Noriyasu Saito, and Nobuyuki Isshiki. 2000. "*In vitro* inhalation behavior of spherically agglomerated steroid particles with carrier lactose." *Advanced Powder Technology* 11 (3):323-332. doi: 10.1163/156855200750172196.

Irngartinger, Meike, V. Camuglia, Michael Damm, J. Goede, and Henderik W. Frijlink. 2004. "Pulmonary delivery of therapeutic peptides via dry powder inhalation: effects of micronisation and manufacturing." *European Journal of Pharmaceutics and Biopharmaceutics* 58 (1):7-14. doi: 10.1016/j.ejpb.2004.03.016.

Jetmalani, Kanika, Paul M Young, T. Smith, Peter J. Stewart, and Daniela Traini. 2012. "Micronized drug powders in binary mixtures and the effect of physical properties on aerosolization from combination drug dry powder inhalers." *Drug Development and Industrial Pharmacy* 38 (12):1504-11. doi: 10.3109/03639045.2012.654793.

Kaialy, Waseem. 2016. "A review of factors affecting electrostatic charging of pharmaceuticals and adhesive mixtures for inhalation." *International Journal of Pharmaceutics* 503 (1-2):262-76. doi: 10.1016/j.ijpharm. 2016.01.076.

Kassem, Nuha Mohammed. 1990. "The influence of carrier surface on the characteristics of inspirable powder aerosls." *Journal of Pharmacy and Pharmacology* 42 (S1):11P-11P. doi: 10.1111/j.2042-7158.1990. tb14384.x.

Kwok, Philip, Amolnat Tunsirikongkon, William Glover, and Hak-Kim Chan. 2011. "Formation of protein nano-matrix particles with controlled surface architecture for respiratory drug delivery." *Pharmaceutical Research* 28 (4):788-796. doi: 10.1007/s11095-010-0332-2.

Lai, Felix K. Y., and John A. Hersey. 1987. "Simulated ordered powder mixture." *International Journal of Pharmaceutics* 36 (2):157-164. doi: 10.1016/0378-5173(87)90151-7.

Leuenberger, Hans Georg W. 2002. "Spray freeze-drying – the process of choice for low water soluble drugs?" *Journal of Nanoparticle Research* 4 (1):111-119. doi: 10.1023/a:1020135603052.

Louey, Margaret D., Sultana Razia, and Peter J. Stewart. 2003. "Influence of physico-chemical carrier properties on the in vitro aerosol deposition from interactive mixtures." *International Journal of Pharmaceutics* 252 (1-2):87-98. doi: 10.1016/S0378-5173(02)00621-X.

Nakpheng, Titpawan, Somchai Sawatdee, Khemmarat Buaking, and Teerapol Srichana. 2011. "Stabilization of luteinizing hormone-releasing hormone in a dry powder formulation and its bioactivity." *Asian Biomedicine* 5 (2):225-233. doi: 10.5372/1905-7415.0502.029.

Park, Chibeom, Ji Eun Park, and Hee Cheul Choi. 2014. "Crystallization-induced properties from morphology-controlled organic crystals." *Accounts of Chemical Research* 47 (8):2353-2364. doi: 10.1021/ ar5000874.

Pilcer, Gabrielle, and Karim Amighi. 2010. "Formulation strategy and use of excipients in pulmonary drug delivery." *International Journal of Pharmaceutics* 392 (1-2):1-19.

Rabinow, Barrett E. 2004. "Nanosuspensions in drug delivery." *Nature Reviews Drug Discovery* 3 (9):785-796. doi: 10.1038/nrd1494.

Rahimpour, Yahya, and Hamed Hamishehkar. 2012. "Lactose engineering for better performance in dry powder inhalers." *Advanced Pharmaceutical Bulletin* 2 (2):183-187. doi: 10.5681/apb.2012.028.

Rahimpour, Yahya, Maryam Kouhsoltani, and Hamed Hamishehkar. 2014. "Alternative carriers in dry powder inhaler formulations." *Drug Discovery Today* 19 (5):618-626. doi: 10.1016/j.drudis.2013.11.013.

Rasenack, Norbert. 2010. "Particle engineering for pulmonary dosage forms." *American Pharmaceutical Review* 13 (3):76-80.

Rasenack, Norbert, and Bernd W. Müller. 2004. "Micron-size drug particles: common and novel micronization techniques." *Pharmaceutical Development and Technology* 9 (1):1-13. doi: 10.1081/pdt-120027417.

Rasenack, Norbert, Hartwig Steckel, and Bernd W. Müller. 2003. "Micronization of anti-inflammatory drugs for pulmonary delivery by a controlled crystallization process." *Journal of Pharmaceutical Sciences* 92 (1):35-44. doi: 10.1002/jps.10274.

Raula, Janne, Anna Lähde, and Esko I. Kauppinen. 2009. "Aerosolization behavior of carrier-free l-leucine coated salbutamol sulphate powders." *International Journal of Pharmaceutics* 365 (1-2):18-25. doi: 10.1016/j.ijpharm.2008.08.017.

Raula, Janne, Jukka Veli Seppälä, Jari E M Malm, Maarit J. Karppinen, and Esko I. Kauppinen. 2012. "Structure and dissolution of l-leucine-coated salbutamol sulphate aerosol particles." *AAPS PharmSciTech* 13 (2):707-712. doi: 10.1208/s12249-012-9789-0.

Rehman, Mohboob, Boris Y. Shekunov, Peter York, David Lechuga-Ballesteros, Danforth P. Miller, Trixie Tan, and Paul Colthorpe. 2004. "Optimisation of powders for pulmonary delivery using supercritical fluid technology." *European Journal of Pharmaceutical Sciences* 22 (1):1-17. doi: 10.1016/j.ejps.2004.02.001.

Rogers, True L., Keith P. Johnston, and Robert O. Williams, 3rd. 2003. "Physical stability of micronized powders produced by spray-freezing into liquid (SFL) to enhance the dissolution of an insoluble drug." *Pharmaceutical Development and Technology* 8 (2):187-97. doi: 10.1081/pdt-120018489.

Saleem, Imran Y., Hugh David C Smyth, and Martin J Telko. 2008. "Prediction of dry powder inhaler formulation performance from surface energetics and blending dynamics." *Drug Development and Industrial Pharmacy* 34 (9):1002-1010.

Sawatdee, Somchai. 2005. "Formulation design of antibuberculosis dry powder inhalers." M.Pharm. Thesis, Faculty of Pharmaceutical Sciences, Prince of Songkla University.

Schiavone, Helena, Srinivas Palakodaty, Andrew R Clark, Peter A. York, and Stelios T. Tzannis. 2004. "Evaluation of SCF-engineered particle-based lactose blends in passive dry powder inhalers." *International Journal of Pharmaceutics* 281 (1-2):55-66. doi: 10.1016/j.ijpharm.2004.05.029.

Shalash, Ahmed O., Abdulla M. Molokhia, and Mustafa M.A. Elsayed. 2015. "Insights into the roles of carrier microstructure in adhesive/carrier-based dry powder inhalation mixtures: Carrier porosity and fine particle content." *European Journal of Pharmaceutics and Biopharmaceutics* 96:291-303. doi: 10.1016/j.ejpb.2015.08.006.

Shekunov, Boris Y., Simon Bristow, Albert H. L. Chow, Lachlan Cranswick, David J. W. Grant, and Peter York. 2003. "Formation of composite crystals by precipitation in supercritical CO2." *Crystal Growth & Design* 3 (4):603-610. doi: 10.1021/cg034026o.

Srichana, Teerapol, Gary P. Martin, and Christopher M. Marriott. 2000. "A human oral-throat cast integrated with a twin-stage impinger for evaluation of dry powder inhalers." *Journal of Pharmacy and Pharmacology* 52 (7):771-778.

Srichana, Teerapol, Roongnapa Suedee, and Wantana Reanmongkol. 2001. "Cyclodextrin as a potential drug carrier in salbutamol dry powder aerosols: The in-vitro deposition and toxicity studies of the complexes." *Respiratory Medicine* 95 (6):513-519. doi: 10.1053/rmed.2001.1079.

Staniforth, John N., John E. Rees, Felix K. Lai, and John A. Hersey. 1982. "Interparticle forces in binary and ternary ordered powder mixes." *Journal of Pharmacy and Pharmacology* 34 (3):141-5.

Steckel, Hartwig, and Heike G. Brandes. 2004. "A novel spray-drying technique to produce low density particles for pulmonary delivery." *International Journal of Pharmaceutics* 278 (1):187-195. doi: 10.1016/j.ijpharm.2004.03.010.

Steckel, Hartwig, and Bernd W. Müller. 1998. "Metered-dose inhaler formulations with beclomethasone-17,21-dipropionate using the ozone friendly propellant R 134a." *European Journal of Pharmaceutics and Biopharmaceutics* 46 (1):77-83.

Steckel, Hartwig, Norbert Rasenack, and Bernd W. Müller. 2003. "In-situ-micronization of disodium cromoglycate for pulmonary delivery." *European Journal of Pharmaceutics and Biopharmaceutics* 55 (2):173-80.

Steckel, Hartwig, Jochen C. Thies, and Bernd W. Müller. 1997. "Micronizing of steroids for pulmonary delivery by supercritical carbon dioxide." *International Journal of Pharmaceutics* 152 (1):99-110. doi: 10.1016/S0378-5173(97)00071-9.

Tabernero, Antonio, Eva M. Martín del Valle, and Miguel A. Galán. 2012. "Supercritical fluids for pharmaceutical particle engineering: Methods, basic fundamentals and modelling." *Chemical Engineering and Processing: Process Intensification* 60:9-25. doi: 10.1016/j.cep. 2012.06.004.

Telko, Martin J., and Anthony J Hickey. 2005. "Dry powder inhaler formulation." *Respiratory Care* 50 (9):1209-1227.

Timsina, M. P., Gary P. Martin, Christopher M. Marriott, David Ganderton, and Michael Yianneskis. 1994. "Drug delivery to the respiratory tract using dry powder inhalers." *International Journal of Pharmaceutics* 101 (1):1-13. doi: 10.1016/0378-5173(94)90070-1.

Vehring, Reinhard. 2008. "Pharmaceutical particle engineering via spray drying." *Pharmaceutical Research* 25 (5):999-1022. doi: 10.1007/s11095-007-9475-1.

Velaga, Sitaram P., Rolf A Berger, and Johan Carlfors. 2002. "Supercritical fluids crystallization of budesonide and flunisolide." *Pharmaceutical Research* 19 (10):1564-71.

Voss, Austin, and Warren H. Finlay. 2002. "Deagglomeration of dry powder pharmaceutical aerosols." *International Journal of Pharmaceutics* 248 (1-2):39-50. doi: 10.1016/S0378-5173(02)00319-8.

Wang, Yajie, Katherine Kho, Wean Sin In Cheow, and Kunn Hadinoto. 2012. "A comparison between spray drying and spray freeze drying for dry powder inhaler formulation of drug-loaded lipid-polymer hybrid nanoparticles." *International Journal of Pharmaceutics* 424 (1-2):98-106. doi: 10.1016/j.ijpharm.2011.12.045.

Weers, Jeffry G., and Danforth P. Miller. 2015. "Formulation design of dry powders for inhalation." *Journal of Pharmaceutical Sciences* 104 (10):3259-3288. doi: 10.1002/jps.24574.

White, Steven, David B. Bennett, Scot Cheu, Patrick W. Conley, Donald B. Guzek, Steven Gray, John Howard, Richard Malcolmson, Joann M. Parker, Phil Roberts, Negar Sadrzadeh, Jacqueline D. Schumacher, Sangita Seshadri, Gregory W. Sluggett, Cynthia L. Stevenson, and Nancy J. Harper. 2005. "EXUBERA®: Pharmaceutical development of a novel product for pulmonary delivery of insulin." *Diabetes Technology & Therapeutics* 7 (6):896-906. doi: 10.1089/dia.2005.7.896.

Wong, Jennifer, Hak-Kim Chan, and Philip Chi Lip Kwok. 2013. "Electrostatics in pharmaceutical aerosols for inhalation." *Therapeutic Delivery* 4 (8):981-1002. doi: 10.4155/tde.13.70.

Xu, Zhen, Heidi M. Mansour, and Anthony J Hickey. 2011. "Particle interactions in dry powder inhaler unit processes: A review." *Journal of Adhesion Science and Technology* 25 (4-5):451-482.

Yadidi, Kambiz. 2016. Dry powder formulations for inhalation. Google Patents.

Young, Paul M, Owen Wood, Jesslynn Ooi, and Daniela Traini. 2011. "The influence of drug loading on formulation structure and aerosol performance in carrier based dry powder inhalers." *International Journal of Pharmaceutics* 416 (1):129-135. doi: 10.1016/j.ijpharm.2011.06.020.

Zanen, Pieter, Liam T. Go, and Jan-Willem J. Lammers. 1994. "The optimal particle size for β-adrenergic aerosols in mild asthmatics." *International Journal of Pharmaceutics* 107 (3):211-217. doi: 10.1016/0378-5173(94)90436-7.

Zeng, Xian Ming, Gary P. Martin, Christopher Marriott, and John N. Pritchard. 2000. "The influence of carrier morphology on drug delivery by dry powder inhalers." *International Journal of Pharmaceutics* 200 (1):93-106.

Zeng, Xian Ming, Gary P. Martin, Seah Kee Tee, Abeer Abu Bu Ghoush, and Christopher Marriott. 1999. "Effects of particle size and adding sequence of fine lactose on the deposition of salbutamol sulphate from a dry powder formulation." *International Journal of Pharmaceutics* 182 (2):133-144. doi: 10.1016/S0378-5173(99)00021-6.

Zhou, Qitony, Li Qu, Thomas R. Gengenbach, Ian C. Larson, Peter J. Stewart, and David A. V. Morton. 2013. "Effect of surface coating with magnesium stearate via mechanical dry powder coating approach on the aerosol performance of micronized drug powders from dry powder inhalers." *AAPS PharmSciTech* 14 (1):38-44. doi: 10.1208/s12249-012-9895-z.

Chapter 5

Excipients and Physical Appearances of Dry Powder Inhalers

5.1. Introduction

Many DPI formulations are comprised of a drug formulated with a range of excipients to produce respirable size for efficient lung delivery. An excipient should be inert and is directed to improve the physical or chemical stability and pharmaceutical properties. The use of an excipient is based on its function(s) in the formulation.

The source of excipients are regulated and approved by the Food and Drug Administration (FDA) and the European Medicines Agency (EMA). These authorities issue regulatory guidance; however, they have no list of excipients for DPIs. Nevertheless, the FDA has a list of materials that are generally recognized as safe. The choice of excipients is based on its potential use in a previously approved product. It is a requirement that the manufacturer of a new dosage form submits full detailed production, safety and toxicology information when applying for new product approval. The number and quantities of excipients incorporated in a formulation should be kept at minimal to obtain regulatory approval.

5.2. Qualified Excipients for Dry Powder Inhaler Formulations

Excipients of currently approved products are summarized in Table 5.1. They have been demonstrated to be safe for use as excipients intended for inhalation.

Table 5.1. Accepted or interesting ingredients for use in DPI formulations. (Adapted from Pilcer and Amighi, International Journal of Pharmaceutics, 392(1-2), 1-19, 2010)

Excipients	Description	Status
Sugars Lactose Glucose Mannitol Trehalose	Coarse/fine carrier	Approved and used Approved (Bronchodual®) Approved (Exubera®) Promising alternative
Phospholipids cholesterol	Used in liposomes, matrix, coating Proliposomes Dry encapsulated material	Biocompatible/biodegradable Antituberculosis (Changsan, Chan, et al. 2009, Changsan, Nilkaeo, et al. 2009, Rojanarat et al. 2011, Rojanarat et al. 2012a, Rojanarat et al. 2012b)
Cholesteryl carbonate esters	Improved drug stability and toxicity and drug bioactivity Dry powder carrier Drug encapsulation materials Controlled release materials	Ongoing laboratory works (Chuealee, Aramwit, and Srichana 2007, Chuealee, Wiedmann, and Srichana 2009, Chuealee et al. 2010, Chuealee et al. 2011, Chuealee, Wiedmann, and Srichana 2011)
Leucine,trileucine	Improved aerosol efficiency Coating on particle surface Carrier Co-carrier with other inert carriers	Endogenous substance but no data on lung toxicity (Rabbani and Seville 2005, Lechuga-Ballesteros et al. 2008, Rattanupatam and Srichana 2014, Kaewjan and Srichana 2016)
Bile salts or their derivatives	Improved drug stability and toxicity Absorption enhancer	Endogenous substances may be accepted but at low dose (2–5% w/w)
	Encapsulated drug material Drug carrier Improve aerosol delivery	(Johansson et al. 2002, Gangadhar, Adhikari, and Srichana 2014, Adhikari et al. 2016, Pilcer and Amighi 2010)

Excipients	Description	Status
Hydroxypropylated -β-CD, natural γ-CD	Drug carrier Host-guest complex Improve aerosol delivery	Promising results (Srichana, Suedee, and Reanmongkol 2001)
Chitosan, trimethyl chitosan	Drug carrier Dimple carriers Improve aerosol delivery Enhance endocytosis to macrophage cells	Promising results but toxic in chronic use (Huang et al. 2005, Grenha et al. 2008, Johansson et al. 2002) Carrier (Ahmad, Nakpheng, and Srichana 2014, Ahmad, Ungphaiboon, and Srichana 2015)
PLGA	Used in sustained release formulations	Immunogenicity observed (Sivadas et al. 2008, Dailey et al. 2006)

5.2.1. Sugars

Lactose is the only carrier in DPIs marketed in the United States. Lactose had long been used as an excipient for oral dosage forms before being deployed in DPIs. Safety and stability profiles of lactose are well established and the manufacturing process concerning the purity and physical properties has been documented. It is easily available and inexpensive. Lactose is highly crystalline with a smooth surface and satisfactory flow properties for a DPI carrier. Lactose is less hygroscopic than other sugars. Several manufacturers offer excipient-grade lactose of various sizes and morphologies. One drawback of lactose is its incompatibility with primary amine moieties. Other sugars, such as mannitol and glucose have been shown to be feasible alternatives to lactose, and it is expected that these sugars will eventually be approved products. Glucose is already used in DPIs in Europe. Mannitol has been used as a pharmaceutical excipient. Its potential use as a carrier in DPI has been reported (Hamishehkar et al. 2010, Steckel and Bolzen 2004). Mannitol is less hygroscopic than lactose and has proven to be the most promising candidate for this application in comparison to the more hygroscopic sugar alcohols such as sorbitol, xylitol, and maltitol. D-Mannitol is currently marketed in some countries as a pulmonary diagnostic DPI (Aridol™) and as a therapeutic dry powder for inhalation for the treatment of cystic fibrosis and chronic bronchitis (Bronchitol™), which were recently approved by the FDA and the European regulatory committee, respectively (Xu et al. 2010). The spherical mannitol in Aridol™ was produced by a spray-drying technique (Tanga et al. 2009). A DPI of ciprofloxacin hydrochloride was prepared by co-spray-drying with different percentages of mannitol. The combined formulation that contained 50% (w/w) mannitol showed the best inhalation performance. It had good stability and the lowest particle cohesion. It was proposed that the co-spray-dried mannitol and ciprofloxacin DPI was an attractive approach to promote mucus clearance in the respiratory tract while simultaneously treating local infections, such as chronic obstructive pulmonary disease and cystic fibrosis (Adi et al. 2010). A high proportion of a fine fraction of the drugs was achieved when mannitol was used as the carrier (Harjunen et al. 2003).

Trehalose dihydrate is a disaccharide and a crystalline hydrate like lactose. Spray-dried inhalable trehalose microparticulate and/or nanoparticulate powders with low water content were successfully produced by spray drying under various conditions and were fully characterized with regard to their water content, morphology and crystallinity (Li and Mansour 2011). A suitable particle size with good dispersibility and solid-state properties of salbutamol sulfate was achieved by co-spray-drying with a trehalose–leucine combination in comparison with other excipients such as mannitol, glycine, and alanine.

Sorbitol can also play a crucial role in the formulation of a respirable protein. Sorbitol can also serve as a stability enhancer during the processing. It was reported that the stability of interferon-β to jet milling was dependent upon the presence of sorbitol in the formulation (Platz, Winters, and Pitt 1994).

5.2.2. Phospholipids and Cholesterol

Phosphatidylcholine and cholesterol have been used in experimental liposomal formulations. Several other materials have been included in experimental DPI formulations with various objectives and varying degree of success. Liposomes are potential drug carriers for a variety of drugs. They entrap a quantity of materials both within their aqueous compartment (for hydrophilic molecules) and within the membrane (for hydrophobic molecules). Liposomes were used to encapsulate rifampicin (RIF) as an alternative formulation for delivery to the respiratory tract (Changsan, Separovic, and Srichana 2008). Factors affecting the stability of liposomes containing RIF were determined. Four liposome suspensions were prepared, containing different millimole ratios of cholesterol (CH) and soybean l-α-phosphatidylcholine (SPC) by the chloroform film method, followed by freeze-drying. Cryo-transmission electron microscopy, photon correlation spectroscopy, ^{2}H and ^{31}P solid-state nuclear magnetic resonance (SSNMR) spectroscopy were used to characterize the liposome suspensions. The obtained liposomes were a mixture of 200–300 nm unilamellar and multilamellar vesicles. A higher CH content in the liposome formulation resulted in a smaller change in the size distribution with time, and a higher CH content was associated with an increase in the ^{2}H-NMR splitting, that was indicative of an increase in the order of the lipid acyl chains. Furthermore, the SSNMR results indicated that RIF was located between the acyl chains of the phospholipid bilayer and was associated with the CH molecules. Fifty percent encapsulation of RIF was obtained when the lipid content was high (SPC 10 mM: CH 10 mM). Mannitol was found to be a suitable cryoprotectant which was attributed to its crystallinity and use of mannitol gave the particles a MMAD of less than 5 μm. Cholesterol does not form a bilayer structure by its own, but it can be incorporated into phospholipid membranes to make major changes in the properties of these membranes and therefore improve the bilayer characteristics of the liposomes (Vemuri and Rhodes 1995). The proliposome was employed to encapsulate several anti-tuberculosis drugs successfully in a dry powder form with good aerosolized properties and acceptable stability (Rojanarat et al. 2011, Rojanarat et al. 2012a, Changsan, Nilkaeo, et al. 2009, Changsan, Chan, et al. 2009). Now the anti-tuberculosis drug is in the clinical trial phase II.

5.2.3. Cholesteryl Carbonate

The cholesterol derivatives were synthesized and employed as a drug carrier for amphotericin B (AmB) for fungal lung infection. It was found that the cholesteryl carbonates had the potential to incorporate AmB into the liquid crystal system. Besides providing aerosolized properties, it also promotes the antifungal activities of AmB (Chuealee et al. 2010, Chuealee, Wiedmann, and Srichana 2011, 2009, Chuealee et al. 2011). The particle size varied inversely to the liquid crystalline content in the cholesteryl carbonate with observed MMADs that ranged from 4 to 8 μm. This was consistent with the visual appearance of the liquid crystals as they possessed low density and were free flowing at room temperature.

5.2.4. Leucine

There are several drug formulations that have included amino acids to improve their aerosolization behavior, decrease the hygroscopicity of a micronized drug, and improve its surface activity and the charge density of cohesive particles (Aquino et al. 2012, Pilcer and Amighi 2010, Seville et al. 2007, Prota et al. 2011). Among the various amino acids used (L-arginine, L-aspartic acid, L-leucine, L-phenylalanine and L-threonine), L-leucine has been shown to be the best excipient in terms of aerosolization (Seville et al. 2007, Chew et al. 2005). It has been suggested that leucine has the best surfactant-like properties (Gliński, Chavepeyer, and Platten 2000) and has the capacity to migrate to the droplet surface during the rapid drying phase of the spray-drying process, and hence the surface characteristics of leucine influence the resultant particle size (Seville et al. 2007). Selection of an appropriate solvent system and an L-leucine concentration will allow for the preparation of a spray-dried powder with enhanced aerosolization properties (Aquino et al. 2012, Rabbani and Seville 2005). Recently our group prepared budesonide co-spray dried with leucine and found no interaction between budesonide and L-leucine. The budesonide dry powders had an aerodynamic diameter of 1.9–2.2 µm at a flow rate of 60 LPM that was suitable for pulmonary delivery (Rattanupatam and Srichana 2014). The incorporation of L-leucine at 10% improved the %FPF by nearly twofold compared to the normal spray-dried pyrazinamide (PZA). Changes in the particle density and morphology were also observed. The dense solid particles of PZA were completely converted to bulk hollow particles with a thin shell by increasing the L-leucine content up to 50% (Kaewjan and Srichana 2016).

5.2.5. Bile Salts and Derivatives

There are many bile salts and derivatives available as absorption enhancers. They have been used for dry powder aerosols (Gangadhar, Adhikari, and Srichana 2014, Adhikari et al. 2016). The main mechanisms behind the absorption enhancement are the production of insulin monomers and an opening of tight junctions between adjacent airway epithelial cells (Johansson et al. 2002). Although the results are very promising, the use of high amounts of bile salts may not be feasible for chronic use since they may damage the epithelial surface. An attempt has been made to enhance the solubility and stability of AmB, and to evaluate its bioactivity and safety for use as an inhaler by using a new excipient, sodium deoxycholate sulfate (SDCS), with the aim of using it as a drug carrier for AmB. Therefore, SDCS was formulated together with AmB as a dry powder by lyophilization. AmB-SDCS was shown to be a potential candidate for the treatment of invasive pulmonary aspergillosis (Gangadhar, Adhikari, and Srichana 2014, Adhikari et al. 2016).

5.2.6. Cyclodextrins and Derivatives

Cyclodextrins (CDs) and their derivatives have been shown to improve the aerosolization properties by modifying the particle morphology and the surface of the drugs (Srichana, Suedee, and Reanmongkol 2001, Ungaro et al. 2006). It can be used not only to enhance the absorption of the drug across the pulmonary epithelium but also to increase the deposition of the drug in rat lungs (Srichana, Suedee, and Reanmongkol 2001). Two types of cyclodextrin were chosen (i.e., γ-cyclodextrin [GCD] and dimethyl-β-cyclodextrin [DMCD]) as carriers in the dry powder formulations. Salbutamol was used as a model drug. The control formulation contained lactose as a carrier. The TSI was used to evaluate the delivery efficiency of these dry powder formulations. The toxicity of the cyclodextrin complexes was investigated in the rat by monitoring the blood urea nitrogen (BUN) and urinary creatinine, as well as determining the hemolysis of human red blood cells. The release of salbutamol from the dry powder formulations was also studied over a period of time. From the results obtained, the formulation containing GCD enhanced the drug delivery to the lower stage of the TSI (deposition=65%) that was much greater than that of both formulations containing DMCD (50%) and the control formulation (40%). After injecting the GCD complex, the BUN and creatinine levels in rats were similar to those obtained in the control while those that received the DMCD complex had higher BUN and creatinine. The hemolysis of red blood cells incubated with the DMCD complex was higher than that obtained with the GCD complex. The drug release in both formulations containing GCD and DMCD was fast (over 70% was released in 5 min) and nearly all the drug was released within 30 min.

5.2.7. Chitosan and Derivatives

Chitosan and trimethyl chitosan which are cationic polysaccharides have also been widely used as absorption enhancers for proteins and peptides. A bioadhesive effect of chitosan particles was observed that might be useful to enhance drug absorption following inhalation. Inhaled chitosan microparticles induced a significant pulmonary inflammatory response in a dose-dependent manner after intratracheal administration (Johansson et al. 2002, Huang et al. 2005, Grenha et al. 2008). The chitosan carrier was spray dried to obtain a spherical shape with a dimpled surface. The chitosan carrier was developed for delivering the antituberculosis drug ethambutol dihydrochloride (EDH) from a DPI to the lungs. The EDH size was 222 nm and the chitosan carrier size was 1.2 µm. The chitosan carrier was spherical in shape with a dimpled surface, and this provided shallow cavities to which the drug was bound, both within its grooves as well as on its surface. The MMAD of the EDH was between 2.3 and 2.7 µm with an FPF of 32-42% of the nominal dose (Ahmad, Nakpheng, and Srichana 2014, Ahmad, Ungphaiboon, and Srichana 2015). The authors suggested that the EDH mixed with a chitosan carrier was suitable for use in a DPI to control tuberculosis.

5.2.8. Poly)Lactic-co-Glycolic Acid(or PLGA

The properties of PLGA have been extensively investigated as a drug carrier for administration via the lung and for sustained drug release. PLGA microspheres have been used in pulmonary delivery for the controlled release of a variety of drugs, including antiasthmatic drugs, antibiotics, peptides and proteins. Due to its extremely slow rate of biodegradation, PLGA is considered unsuitable for pulmonary drug delivery, especially in cases where frequent dosing is required. After inhalation, production of the inflammatory cytokine IL-8 was significantly elevated which indicated its immunogenicity (Dailey et al. 2006, Sivadas et al. 2008). Moreover, the breakdown of PLGA leads to the acidic degradation products such as lactic and glycolic acid that can irritate the lungs.

5.3. Physical Appearances

In a previous chapter, the formulation of a DPI was described together with the production technology. These formulations and technology lead to different product outlooks. For example, large porous particles, nanoporous/microparticles, nanoparticles/microparticles, PulmoSphere®, agglomerates and Trojan microparticles. Table 5.2 lists all of the physical appearances of DPI particles and their advantages.

5.3.1. Large Porous Particles

Large porous particles (LPPs) provide some advantages over conventional microparticles. Inhalation of LPP formulations can prolong drug action in the lungs by reducing the alveolar macrophage phagocytosis rate. There are several preparation techniques of LPPs including a double emulsion approach, precision particle fabrication technology, high-voltage electrostatic antisolvent method, supercritical fluid technology and a single emulsion technique. The preparation techniques for large porous particles are listed in Table 5.3.

Table 5.2. Appearance and advantages of different types of DPI particles

Appearances	Advantages	References
Large porous particles (LPP)	Low alveolar macrophage uptake PLGA microparticles Peptide delivery Proliposomes with low-density	(Koushik et al. 2004, Kwon et al. 2007, Nolan et al. 2009, Yang et al. 2009, Ungaro et al. 2010, Rawat, Majumder, and Ahsan 2008, Meenach et al. 2012, Rojanarat et al. 2012b, Rojanarat et al. 2012a, Dhanda et al. 2013, Steckel and Brandes 2004, Healy et al. 2008, Gupta, Rawat, and Ahsan 2010).
Nanoporous/ microparticles Nanoparticles/ microparticles	Low aggregation High fine particle fraction Nano particle agglomeration	(Nolan et al. 2009, Meenach et al. 2012, Plumley et al. 2009, Ahmad et al. 2012, Healy et al. 2008)
Pulmospheres	Advanced micro/nanospheres specially designed for lung delivery Hollow porous particles Immunoglobulin delivery	(Dellamary et al. 2000, Smith et al. 2001, Duddu et al. 2002, Newhouse et al. 2003, Geller, Weers, and Heuerding 2011, Weers et al. 2015, Hirst et al. 2002, Tarara et al. 2004, Bot et al. 2000)
Solid lipid Nanoparticles	Spherical and hollow with low-density microparticles Peptide and Protein delivery	(Hadinoto et al. 2007, Hadinoto, Zhu, and Tan 2007, Almeida and Souto 2007, Li et al. 2010)
Agglomerates	Particle aggregates with high lung deposition	(Telko and Hickey 2005, Wong et al. 2010)
Trojan microparticles	Targeted to an organ Magnetic nanoparticles Large porous carrier for nanoparticles	(Tewes, Ehrhardt, and Healy 2014, McBride et al. 2013, Upadhyay et al. 2012, Lübbe et al. 1996, Tsapis et al. 2002)
Dimple shapes	Larger surface area Grooves and dimples on surface	(Ahmad, Ungphaiboon, and Srichana 2015, Ahmad, Nakpheng, and Srichana 2014)

Porous microparticles are potential candidates for pulmonary drug delivery. A pore forming agent was employed to obtain porous microparticles. Bernstein et al. (2002) suggested that pore forming agents in the range of 0.01-90% w/v are able to increase the matrix porosity and pore-formation during production. They can be added as solid particles to a polymer solution, to a melted polymer or added as an aqueous solution. Bendroflumethiazide was prepared successfully in porous microparticles by spray drying with ammonium carbonate (Healy et al. 2008). Nolan et al. (2009) prepared nanoporous microparticles of budesonide using ammonium carbonate. Both studies have demonstrated that *in vitro* deposition properties were improved compared to non-porous particles and have the potential use for drug delivery by inhalation. Porous mannitol had the macropores, micropores and nanopores with 3-5 μm in size (Rojanarat et al. 2012a) (Figure 5.1). Ammonium carbonate was observed to produce large hollow particles while ammonium acetate had smaller pores (Figure 5.1b and 5.1d). Nolan et al. (2009) found that a spray drying process could be employed to produce nanoporous budesonide microparticles. The addition of ammonium carbonate was necessary to obtain the porous particles in a methanol/water solvent condition. The density of the porous particles was significantly lower and the surface area significantly higher than that of a non-porous spray-dried preparation. The porous microparticles had improved *in vitro* deposition properties.

Both pore forming agents decomposed when they were heated as shown in equations 5.1 and 5.2. However, in this case, ammonium carbonate decomposed much easier than ammonium acetate and the decomposition yielded ammonia, carbon dioxide, and water.

$$CH_3COONH_4 \xrightarrow{\Delta} CH_3COOH + NH_3 \tag{5.1}$$

$$(NH_4)_2CO_3 \xrightarrow{\Delta} 2NH_3 + CO_2 + H_2O \tag{5.2}$$

Porous mannitol generated by the presence of ammonium carbonate had a higher porosity than that of ammonium acetate because ammonium carbonate decomposed at a lower temperature. It was volatilized more easily than ammonium acetate when heated.

Table 5.3. Preparation of large porous particles and their properties
(Adapted from Healy, A. M. et al.,
Advance Drug Delivery Reviews, 75, 32-52, 2014)

Technique	Porogens	Carrier	Model drug	Properties
Double emulsion	BSA	PLGA	Insulin and VEGF	Initial burst release, sustained for 2 weeks *in vitro*
	PEI	PLGA	LMW heparin	Initial burst release, retain constant rate, increase half-life
	PEI	PLGA	PGE$_1$	increase half-life
	Ammonium bicarbonate	PLGA	Budesonide	Sustained release for 24 h
	Ammonium bicarbonate	PLGA	Doxorubicin	Gradually released over 2 weeks
	SBE-CD	PLGA	Lysozyme	Zero order release up to7 days
	HP-β-CD	PLGA	Insulin	Extended *in vivo* blood glucose control in rats
	HP-β-CD and NaCl	PLGA	Palmityl-acylated exendin-4	Linear release for 5 days, no initial burst
	HP-β-CD and oils	PLGA	Risedronate Sodium	Sustained release up to 15 days
Precision particle fabrication	Oils	PLGA	Ciprofloxacin	Controlled released for 2-4 weeks, *in vitro*
High Voltage electrostatic antisolvent process	Ammonium bicarbonate	PLLA	Methotrexate	Sustained release
SC-CO$_2$	Ammonium bicarbonate	PLLA	Methotrexate	Sustained release
	None	PLGA	Celecoxib	Increased peak level in lungs
Single emulsion	Pluronic F127	PLGA	rhGH	Low initial release, sustained release over 1 month.
Solution Antisolvent Spray drying	Ammonium bicarbonate Ammonium acetate	Mannitol	Pyrazinamide Levofloxacin	High fine particle fraction Low macrophage uptake

*BSA = bovine serum albumin, PEI = polyethyleneimine, PLGA = poly (lactic-co-glycolic acid), SBE-β-CD = sulfobutylether β-cyclodextrin, SC-CO$_2$ = supercritical carbon dioxide

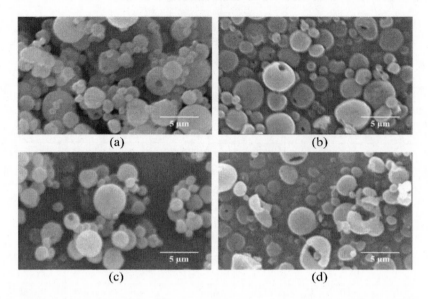

(a)   (b)

(c)   (d)

Figure 5.1. The SEM images of porous mannitol generated with ammonium acetate (a-b) and with ammonium carbonate (c-d) (bar = 5 μm).

The PLGA LPPs of doxorubicin hydrochloride was prepared by adding ammonium bicarbonate to an aqueous internal phase (primary phase) prior to mixing with the secondary aqueous phase (Yang et al. 2009). Particles presented with MMADs of 4.6-5.7 μm and with FPFs of 16-34%. These particles were able to reduce macrophage uptake and prolong drug release. Ungaro et al. (2010) applied LPPs to load rhodamine B isothiocyanate–dextran. These LPPs were considered to be gas-foamed LPPs. During the production, ammonium bicarbonate released ammonia and the carbon dioxide gasses resulted in pore formation in the prepared particles. The LPPs showed favorable *in vitro* and *in vivo* deposition in rats. Gupta et al. (2010) reported the double emulsion solvent evaporation of PLGA LPPs by incorporating prostaglandin E_1 (PGE$_1$) in the external phase. Particle MMADs varied from 1 to 4 μm and showed a prolonged release of PGE$_1$ after pulmonary administration. Later, Gupta and Ahsan (2011) reported a modified approach to PLGA-PGE$_1$ LPP production where the drug was incorporated into the aqueous internal phase by solubilization in a small quantity of ethanol. The aqueous internal phase was also supplemented with polyethyleneimine (PEI) as a pore forming agent and a drug-loading enhancer (Figure 5.2). All reported MMADs were below 5 μm (Gupta and Ahsan 2011).

The double emulsion solvent evaporation method is the most widely exploited method to prepare LPPs. PLGA is commonly used as the carrier material for LPPs. The porogens such as ammonium bicarbonate, HP-β-CD and sodium chloride were added during the preparation process (Table 5.3). This method is suitable for encapsulating water-soluble hydrophilic drugs such as proteins and peptides. The porogens were broken down into gas bubbles during the emulsification process to form the porous matrix.

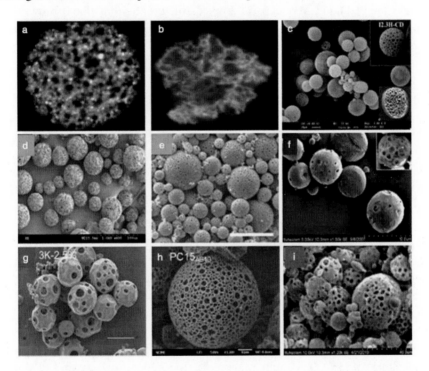

Figure 5.2. Scanning electron micrographs of (a) polylactide glycolide, (b) poly(lactic acid-co-lysine-graft-lysine), (c) b, (d) bovine serum albumin, (e) camptothecin, (f) low molecular weight heparin-PLGA-polyethylene imine, (g) double emulsion solvent evaporation ammonium bicarbonate–PLGA-Placebo, (h) DOTAP, (i) prostaglandin E_1-PLGA-PEI large porous particles. (Reprinted from Healy, A. M. et al., Advanced Drug Delivery Reviews, 75, 32-52, 2014. With permission from Elsevier).

The LPPs developed by Ungaro et al. (2010), Kwon et al. (2007), Rawat et al. (2008) and Meenach et al. (2012) presented MMAD values of 3-17 μm with a high FPF and emitted doses, and extended release profiles. Figure 5.2 shows the SEM images of the LPPs with various porogens, carrier materials and active pharmaceutical ingredients. PEI is also a suitable pore forming agent for the conventional double emulsion solvent evaporation production process. It markedly increased the porosity of the LPPs (Rawat, Majumder, and Ahsan 2008). The osmotic pressure imbalance between the internal and external aqueous phases may contribute to the formation of porosity. On the other hand, electrostatic charge interactions between the negatively charged low molecular weight heparin (LMW heparin) and PEI played an important role in the pore formation process because they increased the entrapment of water in the PEI and LMW heparin droplet structure. Sublimation of water that was entrapped in the droplet structure during lyophilization resulted in large pores in the particles.

5.3.2. Modified Production Processes for Large Porous Particles

Steckel and Brandes (2004) expanded the conventional approach to solution or suspension spray drying for the production of LPPs. LPPs of salbutamol sulfate were produced by spray drying of a compressed emulsion. The emulsion was composed of an oil phase (propellant: Solkane™227) and an aqueous phase containing salbutamol sulfate, phosphatidylcholine, poloxamer 188, calcium chloride and HP-β-CD. Koushik et al. (2004) prepared deslorelin-PLGA-HP-β-CD LPPs using a SC-CO$_2$. PLGA in the methylene chloride was combined with a methanolic solution of deslorelin with or without HP-β-CD to produce the oil phase. Then the oil phase was dispersed in an aqueous phase of polyvinyl acetate. The formed microparticles were centrifuged, washed and freeze-dried. They were subsequently suspended in SC-CO$_2$. SCF processing was able to produce LPPs using a low process temperature of 33°C. A similar approach to produce celecoxib LPPs was reported by Dhanda et al. (2013). PLGA microparticles were produced by homogenization of the primary emulsion followed by solvent evaporation. The oil phase was composed of celecoxib, PLGA and dichloromethane and the aqueous phase of polyvinyl acetate. The primary emulsion was subsequently diluted with the aqueous solution and stirred to evaporate the dichloromethane. Microparticles were isolated, washed, freeze-dried and reprocessed using SC-CO$_2$ to produce LPPs. Celecoxib–PLGA LPPs were proven to have better control of drug levels in the lungs and improved the lung accumulation index following a single administration compared to conventional non-porous particles.

5.3.3. Nanoporous/Nanoparticulate Microparticles

Nanoporous/nanoparticulate microparticles (NPMPs) were introduced by Healy at al. (2008). The production of excipient-free porous microparticles by spray drying was obtained by a mixed solvent/antisolvent system. The SEM of NPMPs of bendroflumethiazide, budesonide, p-aminosalicylic acid, sodium cromoglycate, ambroxol HCl and raffinose are shown in Figure 5.3.

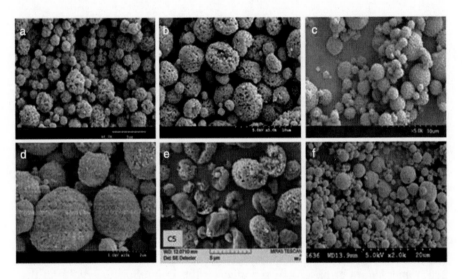

Figure 5.3 .Scanning electron micrographs of selected NPMPs materials: (a) bendroflumethiazide; (b) budesonide; (c) p-aminosalicylic acid (PAS); (d) sodium cromoglycate; (e) budesonide ambroxol HCl; (f) raffinose. (Reprinted from Healy, A. M. et al., Advanced Drug Delivery Reviews, 75, 32-52, 2014. With permission from Elsevier).

A different co-solvent system (ethanol/water and methanol/water) was also used in the NPMP production for hydrophobic drug and excipients. In contrast, the water/methanol/butyl acetate and methanol/butyl acetate were suitable for more hydrophilic materials. During the atomization of the spray drying process, droplets were formed and rapid drying of these droplets occurred on contact with the warm drying gas. The solubility of the solute may condense out as a nanosized liquid phase within the droplet. As further solvent loss occurs, the solute phase droplets come closer together, and the solute may precipitate out as primary nanoparticles leading to the formation of NPMP. All NPMPs produced particle sizes of about 3 μm and due to their porous nature the NPMPs had lower bulk densities than the spray dried non-porous particles.

NPMPs were all amorphous in nature with the exception of PAS NPMPs that were crystalline. The NPMPs improved the FPFs to 50–80% when compared to the non-porous particles. The improved aerosolization properties of the NPMPs may be attributed to the reduced interparticulate contact.

5.3.4. PulmoSphere®

SD became the main process for the production of the PulmoSphere® (Weers et al. 2015). PulmoSphere® microparticles are generated from an emulsion-based feed. The PulmoSphere® particles are less than 5 μm in size. The porous particles have reduced particle–particle interaction and cohesion, and the porous nature of the particles has improved flowability and aerosolization. Dellamary et al. (2000) produced PulmoSphere® containing cromolyn sodium, salbutamol sulfate or formoterol fumarate in a preparation of an emulsion containing the drug and additives in an aqueous solution. The dispersed phase was composed of fluorocarbon Perflubron™, while the aqueous phase contained the emulsifier (e.g., phosphatidylcholine). The homogenized oil-in-water (o/w) emulsion was mixed with the aqueous solutions and spray dried. During SD, a solid phase was separated from the evaporating solvent. The fluorocarbon evaporated from the particle surface that acted as a pore-former. Bot et al. (2000), Smith et al. (2001), Hirst et al. (2002) and Tarara et al. (2004) reported on the PulmoSphere® platform that produced particles using hIgG, gentamicin sulfate, salbutamol sulfate and budesonide, respectively.

Duddu et al. (2002) modified the PulmoSphere® for DPIs. In contrast to previous work, budesonide was a microcrystalline form instead of being dissolved in an aqueous solution. First, microcrystals were combined with a prepared emulsion of perflubron in water. Second, the suspension-emulsion was homogenized with an aqueous solution of calcium chloride with lactose monohydrate and spray dried. The PulmoSphere® can be formulated in either DPIs or pMDIs (Figure 5.4). Pulmonary deposition of the budesonide PulmoSphere® was around 60%. The peak plasma budesonide for the PulmoSphere® was about two times greater than for the Pulmicort®. The t_{max} was observed at 5 min for the PulmoSphere® compared to 20 min for the Pulmicort®.

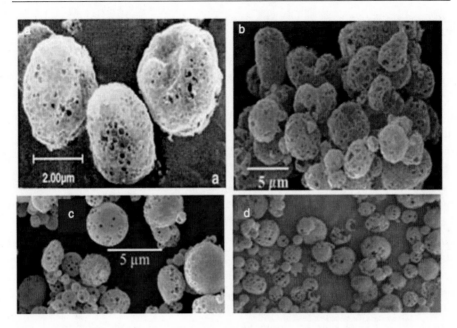

Figure 5.4. Scanning electron micrographs of PulmoSphere®: (a) sodium cromoglycate; (b) budesonide as DPIs; (c) budesonide as pMDIs; (d) tobramycin as DPIs. (Reprinted from Healy, A. M. et al., Advanced Drug Delivery Reviews, 75, 32-52, 2014. With permission from Elsevier).

Newhouse et al. (2003) compared tobramycin PulmoSphere® inhaled through a Turbospin® to a nebulized tobramycin (TOBI®). Whole-lung deposition of the PulmoSphere® was around 34% compared to 5% for the TOBI®. Peak plasma tobramycin for PulmoSphere® was about three times larger than the TOBI®. While the area under the curve (AUC) was about two times greater. Geller et al. (2011) reported an encapsulated tobramycin PulmoSphere® (Figure 5.4) inhaled through a Podhaler™. This was compared to a 300 mg tobramycin solution for inhalation. Serum tobramycin levels were found to be similar for both preparations. The FDA approved the TOBI®Podhaler™ to treat a bacterial lung infection in cystic fibrosis in 2013.

Weers et al. (2015) investigated dose emission of placebo PulmoSphere® particles administered as dry powders with a portable, blister-based Simoon DPI. *In vitro* particle depositions were found to be independent on the inhalation maneuver.

5.3.5. Solid Lipid Nanoparticles

The application of polymeric colloidal drug carriers in pulmonary formulations is often limited by the unknown toxicity of the carrier in the lungs. Even biodegradable polymers have not yet undergone any rigorous toxicity testing for safe delivery via the lungs. It has been suggested that lipids have a faster biodegradation and higher tolerability in the lungs compared to particles from polymeric materials. It is feasible that aqueous suspensions and solid lipid dry powders can be used for pulmonary administration. Lipid carriers include liposomes, lipid emulsions, lipid complexes and solid lipid micro- and nanoparticles (SLN). One of the common methods for preparing SLN is high-pressure homogenization. The drug is dissolved in a molten lipid and then homogenized in an aqueous medium into 200-500 nm particle sizes followed by solidification. This method follows the same processing steps as the lipid emulsions which is a well-established pharmaceutical manufacturing process and can be easily scaled-up. The major drawback, however, is the limited drug solubility in the molten lipid and the solidified lipid phase. Alternatively, SLN can be prepared by precipitation from o/w emulsions which may produce a smaller particle size with a higher drug loading. This can also be accomplished as a continuous process using a supercritical fluid extraction method as detailed previously.

5.3.6. Agglomerates

Suspensions of micronized drug crystals and nanoparticles are spray-dried to form particulate aggregates. Inhalable particles of water-insoluble drugs and/or porous or hollow particles are able to improve the aerodynamic properties of the particles. The aggregates consisted of crystals dispersed in a matrix of amorphous excipients. Different degrees of drug crystallinity can be obtained depending on the engineered particles in the suspensions and the SD conditions. This technique was employed to prepare corticosteroid, disodium cromoglycate and chitosan nanoparticles. Porous aggregates of budesonide and albuterol sulfate were prepared using the PulmoSphere® platform. These particles had improved in physical stability, content uniformity and aerosolization efficiency compared to conventional micronized materials. Amorphous solid dispersions of poorly soluble drugs can be prepared by conventional and modified SD. Drug particles can be co-spray dried with nanospheres of hydrophilic polymers to modify the particle surface and to enhance dispersion.

5.3.7. Trojan Microparticles/Magnetically Targeted Dry Powder Aerosols

Magnetization as a means of targeting drugs to the lungs was investigated. Magnetization involves incorporating magnetically active particles to a chemotherapeutic drug. Such particles can be guided to a specific location in the body using a strong external magnet. Lübbe et al. (1996) performed the first clinical trials for epirubicin to treat breast cancer by magnetic carriers. Epirubicin was ionically bound to a modified carbohydrate layer on iron-oxide nanoparticles (Upadhyay et al. 2012). They observed the accumulation of nanoparticles in the target area after exposure to the magnetic field. A release of heat to the surrounding tissues contributed to tumor cell death through hyperthermia (Upadhyay et al. 2012). The lipid system presented thermo-sensitive characteristics of drug release at hyperthermic conditions (45°C). Superparamagnetic iron oxide nanoparticles (SPION) loaded lipid system produced an inhalable FPF of 30% using an Aerosolizer^{TM}.

Tewes et al. (2014) prepared SPIONs-loaded Trojan microparticles by spray drying. The resulting particles delivered by a Handihaler® were spherical with a porous surface and an MMAD of 2.2 ± 0.8 μm. In the presence of a magnetic field, the lower stage deposition increased significantly. These Trojan particles were highly sensitive to the magnetic field. The authors suggested that these particles would be useful to treat localized lung disease such as cancer or bacterial infection. McBride et al. (2013) prepared magnetically SPION-loaded Trojan microparticles as a dry powder nano-in-microparticles (NIMs). The NIMs were prepared from a suspension of lactose, doxorubicin and Fe_3O_4 SPIONs by SD. TEM and SEM micrographs demonstrated the porous nature of the NIMs and the surface localization of SPIONs. Deposition of the NIMs was performed to mimic the conducting airway deposition. This *in vitro* study demonstrated more than twice the spatial deposition and retention of NIMs, compared to a liquid suspension.

Tsapis et al. (2002) spray dried three different systems to produce Trojan microparticles: (1) polystyrene nanoparticles in ethanol/water (7:3 v/v) containing dipalmitoylphosphatidylcholine, 1,2-dimyristoyl-sn-glycero-3-phosphoethanol-amine and lactose with or without hydroxypropyl cellulose; (2) silica nanoparticles were added to (1), except that water was replaced by 25 mM Tris buffer (pH 9.25) and (3) polystyrene nanoparticles were added to bovine serum albumin in phosphate buffer with the addition of ammonium bicarbonate. The nanoparticles were used to prepare the Trojan particles of 25-100 nm (Figure 5.5).

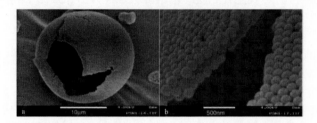

Figure 5.5. Polystyrene-DPPC Trojan particles: (a) typical hollow sphere Trojan particles observed from the spray drying of a solution of polystyrene nanoparticles (170 nm); (b) a magnified view of the particle's surface. (Reprinted from Tsapis, N. et al., Proceedings of the National Academy of Sciences, 99(19), 12001-12005, 2002. Copyright (2002) National Academy of Sciences, U.S.A.).

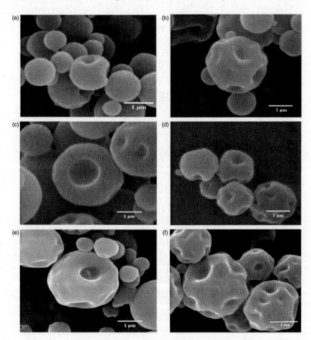

Figure 5.6. SEM images of chitosan particles that were taken from spraying of a chitosan solution at 150 °C with a feeding rate of 3 mL/min. (Reprinted from Ahmad, M. I. et al., Drug Development and Industrial Pharmacy, 41(5), 791-800, 2015. With permission from Taylor & Francis).

These Trojan microparticles exhibited a much better flow and aerosolization properties than the typical nanoparticles (NPs). The NPs were held together in the Trojan particles by van der Waals forces within a matrix of added ingredients such as biopolymers or phospholipids.

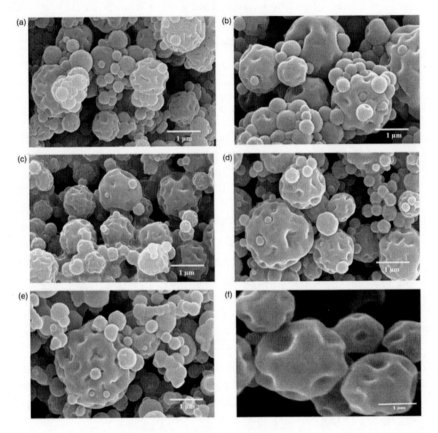

Figure 5.7. The SEM images of chitosan and ethambutol mixtures of 1:2 (a), 1:2.5 (b), 1:3.3 (c), 1: 5 (d), 1:10 (e) weight ratios and carrier alone (f). (Reprinted from Ahmad, M. I. et al., Drug Development and Industrial Pharmacy, 41(5), 791-800, 2015. With permission from Taylor & Francis).

5.3.8. Dimple Shaped Carriers

Dimple-shaped chitosan particles were prepared for use as a carrier for ethambutol. The dimple shape of the chitosan carrier provided grooves over its whole surface that provided a good space for a drug to bind and help in its dispersion in the oral cavities. Hence, a dimple-shaped carrier is likely to have better aerosolization properties (Ahmad, Ungphaiboon, and Srichana 2015, Ahmad, Nakpheng, and Srichana 2014). Figure 5.6 shows the dimple chitosan prepared with different conditions to generate dimples on the surface of the carrier. Figure 5.7 shows the nanosized drug particle after mixing with the dimple shaped carrier. It was found that the drug particles would sit in the grooves rather than on the smooth surface.

References

Adhikari, Kajiram, Wilaiporn Buatong, Ekawat Thawithong, Tan Suwandecha, and Teerapol Srichana. 2016. "Factors affecting enhanced permeation of amphotericin B across cell membranes and safety of formulation." *AAPS PharmSciTech* 17 (4):820-828. doi: 10.1208/s12249-015-0406-x.

Adi, Handoko, Paul M Young, Hak-Kim Chan, Helen Agus, and Daniela Traini. 2010. "Co-spray-dried mannitol–ciprofloxacin dry powder inhaler formulation for cystic fibrosis and chronic obstructive pulmonary disease." *European Journal of Pharmaceutical Sciences* 40 (3):239-247.

Ahmad, Md Iftekhar, Titpawan Nakpheng, and Teerapol Srichana. 2014. "The safety of ethambutol dihydrochloride dry powder formulations containing chitosan for the possibility of treating lung tuberculosis." *Inhalation Toxicology* 26 (14):908-917.

Ahmad, Md Iftekhar, Suwipa Ungphaiboon, and Teerapol Srichana. 2015. "The development of dimple-shaped chitosan carrier for ethambutol dihydrochloride dry powder inhaler." *Drug Development and Industrial Pharmacy* 41 (5):791-800.

Ahmad, Sana, Bernard Jousseaume, Thierry Toupance, Odile Babot, Guy Campet, Christine Labrugere, Joachim Brotz, and Ulrike Kunz. 2012. "A new route towards nanoporous TiO2 as powders or thin films from the thermal treatment of titanium-based hybrid materials." *Dalton Transactions* 41 (1):292-299. doi: 10.1039/C1DT11087J.

Almeida, António J., and Eliana Souto. 2007. "Solid lipid nanoparticles as a drug delivery system for peptides and proteins." *Advanced Drug Delivery Reviews* 59 (6):478-490. doi: 10.1016/j.addr.2007.04.007.

Aquino, Rita Patrizia Atrizia, Lucia Prota, Giulia Auriemma, Antonietta Santoro, Teresa Mencherini, Gaia Colombo, and Paola F. Russo. 2012. "Dry powder inhalers of gentamicin and leucine: formulation parameters, aerosol performance and in vitro toxicity on CuFi1 cells." *International Journal of Pharmaceutics* 426 (1–2):100-107. doi: 10.1016/j.ijpharm. 2012.01.026.

Bernstein, Howard, Donald Chickering, Sarwat Khattak, and Julie Straub. 2002. Matrices formed of polymer and hydrophobic compounds for use in drug delivery. Acusphere, Inc.

Bot, Adrian I, Thomas E Tarara, Dan J Smith, Simona R Bot, Catherine M Woods, and Jeffry G Weers. 2000. "Novel lipid-based hollow-porous microparticles as a platform for immunoglobulin delivery to the respiratory tract." *Pharmaceutical Research* 17 (3):275-283.

Changsan, Narumon, Hak-Kim Chan, Frances Separovic, and Teerapol Srichana. 2009. "Physicochemical characterization and stability of rifampicin liposome dry powder formulations for inhalation." *Journal of Pharmaceutical Sciences* 98 (2):628-639. doi: 10.1002/jps.21441.

Changsan, Narumon, Athip Nilkaeo, Pethchawan Pungrassami, and Teerapol Srichana. 2009. "Monitoring safety of liposomes containing rifampicin on respiratory cell lines and in vitro efficacy against Mycobacterium bovis in alveolar macrophages." *Journal of Drug Targeting* 17 (10):751-762. doi: 10.3109/10611860903079462.

Changsan, Narumon, Frances Separovic, and Teerapol Srichana. 2008. "Determination of rifampicin location in cholesterol-lipid liposomes by 2H and 31P solid-state NMR." 2008 2nd IEEE International Nanoelectronics Conference, INEC 2008.

Chew, Nora Y. K., Boris Yu Shekunov, Henry H. Y. Tong, Albert H. L. Chow, Charles Savage, James Wu, and Hak-Kim Chan. 2005. "Effect of amino acids on the dispersion of disodium cromoglycate powders." *Journal of Pharmaceutical Sciences* 94 (10):2289-2300. doi: 10.1002/jps.20426.

Chuealee, Rabkwan, Pornanong Aramwit, Kusumarn Noipha, and Teerapol Srichana. 2011. "Bioactivity and toxicity studies of amphotericin B incorporated in liquid crystals." *European Journal of Pharmaceutical Sciences* 43 (4):308-317. doi: 10.1016/j.ejps.2011.05.009.

Chuealee, Rabkwan, Pornanong Aramwit, and Teerapol Srichana. 2007. "Characteristics of cholesteryl cetyl carbonate liquid crystals as drug delivery systems." Proceedings of the 2nd IEEE International Conference on Nano/Micro Engineered and Molecular Systems, IEEE NEMS 2007.

Chuealee, Rabkwan, Timothy Scott Wiedmann, and Teerapol Srichana. 2009. "Thermotropic behavior of sodium cholesteryl carbonate." *Journal of Materials Research* 24 (1):156-163. doi: 10.1557/jmr.2009.0027.

Chuealee, Rabkwan, Timothy Scott Wiedmann, and Teerapol Srichana. 2011. "Physicochemical properties and antifungal activity of amphotericin b incorporated in cholesteryl carbonate esters." *Journal of Pharmaceutical Sciences* 100 (5):1727-1735. doi: 10.1002/jps.22398.

Chuealee, Rabkwan, Timothy Scott Wiedmann, Roongnapa Suedee, and Teerapol Srichana. 2010. "Interaction of Amphotericin B with cholesteryl palmityl carbonate ester." *Journal of Pharmaceutical Sciences* 99 (11):4593-4602. doi: 10.1002/jps.22176.

Dailey, Lea Ann Nn, Norman Jekel, Ludger Fink, Tobias Gessler, Thomas Schmehl, Matthias Wittmar, Thomas H. Kissel, and Wernar Seeger. 2006. "Investigation of the proinflammatory potential of biodegradable nanoparticle drug delivery systems in the lung." *Toxicology and Applied Pharmacology* 215 (1):100-108. doi: 10.1016/j.taap.2006.01.016.

Dellamary, Luis A., Thomas E. Tarara, Dan J. Smith, Christopher H. Woelk, Anastasios Adractas, Michael L. Costello, Howard Gill, and Jeffry G. Weers. 2000. "Hollow porous particles in metered dose inhalers." *Pharmaceutical Research* 17 (2):168-174. doi: 10.1023/a:10075 13213292.

Dhanda, Devender S., Puneet Tyagi, Sidney S. Mirvish, and Uday B. Kompella. 2013. "Supercritical fluid technology based large porous celecoxib–PLGA microparticles do not induce pulmonary fibrosis and sustain drug delivery and efficacy for several weeks following a single dose." *Journal of Controlled Release* 168 (3):239-250. doi: 10.1016/j.jconrel.2013.03.027.

Duddu, Sarma P., Steven A. Sisk, Yulia H. Walter, Thomas E. Tarara, Kevin R. Trimble, Andrew R. Clark, Michael A. Eldon, Rebecca C. Elton, Matthew Pickford, Peter H. Hirst, Stephen P. Newman, and Jeffry G. Weers. 2002. "Improved lung delivery from a passive dry powder inhaler using an engineered PulmoSphere® powder." *Pharmaceutical Research* 19 (5):689-695. doi: 10.1023/a:1015322616613.

Gangadhar, Katkam N., Kajiram Adhikari, and Teerapol Srichana. 2014. "Synthesis and evaluation of sodium deoxycholate sulfate as a lipid drug carrier to enhance the solubility, stability and safety of an amphotericin B inhalation formulation." *International Journal of Pharmaceutics* 471 (1-2):430-438. doi: 10.1016/j.ijpharm.2014.05.066.

Geller, David E, Jeffry Weers, and Silvia Heuerding. 2011. "Development of an inhaled dry-powder formulation of tobramycin using PulmoSphere™ technology." *Journal of Aerosol Medicine and Pulmonary Drug Delivery* 24 (4):175-182.

Gliński, Jacek, Guy Chavepeyer, and Jean-Karl Platten. 2000. "Surface properties of aqueous solutions of L-leucine." *Biophysical Chemistry* 84 (2):99-103.

Grenha, Ana, Carmen Remuñán-López, Edison LS Carvalho, and Begona Seijo. 2008. "Microspheres containing lipid/chitosan nanoparticles complexes for pulmonary delivery of therapeutic proteins." *European Journal of Pharmaceutics and Biopharmaceutics* 69 (1):83-93.

Gupta, Vivek, and Fakhrul Ahsan. 2011. "Influence of PEI as a core modifying agent on PLGA microspheres of PGE1, a pulmonary selective vasodilator." *International Journal of Pharmaceutics* 413 (1–2):51-62. doi: 10.1016/j.ijpharm.2011.04.017.

Gupta, Vivek, Amit Rawat, and Fakhrul Ahsan. 2010. "Feasibility study of aerosolized prostaglandin E1 microspheres as a noninvasive therapy for pulmonary arterial hypertension." *Journal of Pharmaceutical Sciences* 99 (4):1774-1789.

Hadinoto, Kunn, Ponpan Phanapavudhikul, Zhu Kewu, and Reginald B. H. Tan. 2007. "Dry powder aerosol delivery of large hollow nanoparticulate aggregates as prospective carriers of nanoparticulate drugs: Effects of phospholipids." *International Journal of Pharmaceutics* 333 (1-2):187-198. doi: 10.1016/j.ijpharm.2006.10.009.

Hadinoto, Kunn, Kewu Zhu, and Reginald B. H. Tan. 2007. "Drug release study of large hollow nanoparticulate aggregates carrier particles for pulmonary delivery." *International Journal of Pharmaceutics* 341 (1-2):195-206. doi: 10.1016/j.ijpharm.2007.03.035.

Hamishehkar, Hamed, Jaber Emami, Abdolhossein Rouholamini Najafabadi, Kambiz Gilani, Mohsen Minaiyan, Hamid Mahdavi, and Ali Nokhodchi. 2010. "Effect of carrier morphology and surface characteristics on the development of respirable PLGA microcapsules for sustained-release pulmonary delivery of insulin." *International Journal of Pharmaceutics* 389 (1-2):74-85. doi: 10.1016/j.ijpharm.2010.01.021.

Harjunen, Päivi, Tapio Lankinen, Heikki Salonen, Vesa-Pekka Lehto, and Kristiina Järvinen. 2003. "Effects of carriers and storage of formulation on the lung deposition of a hydrophobic and hydrophilic drug from a DPI." *International Journal of Pharmaceutics* 263 (1):151-163.

Healy, Anne Marie, Maria Ines Nes Amaro, Krzystof Jan An Paluch, and Lidia Tajber. 2014. "Dry powders for oral inhalation free of lactose carrier particles." *Advanced Drug Delivery Reviews* 75:32-52. doi: 10.1016/ j.addr.2014.04.005.

Healy, Anne Marie, Bernard F. McDonald, Lidia Tajber, and Owen I. Corrigan. 2008. "Characterisation of excipient-free nanoporous microparticles (NPMPs) of bendroflumethiazide." *European Journal of Pharmaceutics and Biopharmaceutics* 69 (3):1182-1186. doi: 10.1016/ j.ejpb.2008.04.020.

Hirst, Peter H., Gary R. Pitcairn, Jeff G. Weers, Thomas E. Tarara, Andrew R. Clark, Luis A. Dellamary, Gail Hall, Jolene Shorr, and Stephen P. Newman. 2002. "*In vivo* Lung deposition of hollow porous particles from a pressurized metered dose inhaler." *Pharmaceutical Research* 19 (3):258-264. doi: 10.1023/a:1014482615914.

Huang, Min, Chee-Wai Fong, Eugene Khor, and Lee-Yong Lim. 2005. "Transfection efficiency of chitosan vectors: effect of polymer molecular weight and degree of deacetylation." *Journal of Controlled Release* 106 (3):391-406.

Johansson, Fredrik I., Elisabeth Hjertberg, Stefan J. Eirefelt, Ann Tronde, and Ursula Hultkvist Bengtsson. 2002. "Mechanisms for absorption enhancement of inhaled insulin by sodium taurocholate." *European Journal of Pharmaceutical Sciences* 17 (1-2):63-71.

Kaewjan, Kanogwan, and Teerapol Srichana. 2016. "Nano spray-dried pyrazinamide-l-leucine dry powders, physical properties and feasibility used as dry powder aerosols." *Pharmaceutical Development and Technology* 21 (1):68-75. doi: 10.3109/10837450.2014.971373.

Koushik, Kavitha, Devender S. Dhanda, Narayan P. S. Cheruvu, and Uday B. Kompella. 2004. "Pulmonary delivery of deslorelin: Large-porous PLGA particles and HP-β-CD complexes." *Pharmaceutical Research* 21 (7):1119-1126. doi: 10.1023/b:pham.0000032997.96823.88.

Kwon, Min Jung, Jun Ho Bae, Jung Ju Kim, Kun Na, and Eun Seong Lee. 2007. "Long acting porous microparticle for pulmonary protein delivery." *International Journal of Pharmaceutics* 333 (1–2):5-9. doi: 10.1016/ j.ijpharm.2007.01.016.

Lechuga-Ballesteros, David, Chatan Charan, Cheryl L M Stults, Cynthia L. Stevenson, Danforth P. Miller, Reinhard Vehring, Vathana Tep, and Mei Chang Kuo. 2008. "Trileucine improves aerosol performance and stability of spray-dried powders for inhalation." *Journal of Pharmaceutical Sciences* 97 (1):287-302. doi: 10.1002/jps.21078.

Li, Xiaojian, and Heidi M Mansour. 2011. "Physicochemical characterization and water vapor sorption of organic solution advanced spray-dried inhalable trehalose microparticles and nanoparticles for targeted dry powder pulmonary inhalation delivery." *AAPS PharmSciTech* 12 (4):1420-1430.

Li, Yan-Zhen, Xun Sun, Tao Gong, Jie Liu, Jiao Zuo, and Zhi-Rong Zhang. 2010. "Inhalable microparticles as carriers for pulmonary delivery of thymopentin-loaded solid lipid nanoparticles." *Pharmaceutical Research* 27 (9):1977-1986. doi: 10.1007/s11095-010-0201-z.

Lübbe, Andreas Stephan, Christian Bergemann, Winfried Huhnt, Thomas Fricke, Hanno Riess, Jeffery Walter Brock, and Dieter Huhn. 1996. "Preclinical experiences with magnetic drug targeting: tolerance and efficacy." *Cancer Research* 56 (20):4694-4701.

McBride, Amber A., Dominique N. Price, Loreen R. Lamoureux, Alaa A. Elmaoued, Jose M. Vargas, Natalie L. Adolphi, and Pavan Muttil. 2013. "Preparation and characterization of novel magnetic nano-in-microparticles for site-specific pulmonary drug delivery." *Molecular Pharmaceutics* 10 (10):3574-3581. doi: 10.1021/mp3007264.

Meenach, Samantha A., Yu Jeong Kim, Kevin J. Kauffman, Naveen Kanthamneni, Eric M. Bachelder, and Kristy M. Ainslie. 2012. "Synthesis, optimization, and characterization of camptothecin-loaded acetalated dextran porous microparticles for pulmonary delivery." *Molecular Pharmaceutics* 9 (2):290-298. doi: 10.1021/mp2003785.

Newhouse, Michael T, Peter H Hirst, Sarma P Duddu, Yulia H Walter, Thomas E Tarara, Andrew R Clark, and Jeffry G Weers. 2003. "Inhalation of a dry powder tobramycin PulmoSphere formulation in healthy volunteers." *Chest Journal* 124 (1):360-366.

Nolan, Lorraine M., Lidia Tajber, Bernard F. McDonald, Ahmad S. Barham, Owen I. Corrigan, and Anne Marie Healy. 2009. "Excipient-free nanoporous microparticles of budesonide for pulmonary delivery." *European Journal of Pharmaceutical Sciences* 37 (5):593-602. doi: 10.1016/j.ejps.2009.05.007.

Pilcer, Gabrielle, and Karim Amighi. 2010. "Formulation strategy and use of excipients in pulmonary drug delivery." *International Journal of Pharmaceutics* 392 (1–2):1-19. doi: 10.1016/j.ijpharm.2010.03.017.

Platz, Robert M, Mark A Winters, and Colin G Pitt. 1994. Pulmonary administration of granulocyte colony stimulating factor. Amgen Inc.

Plumley, Carl, Eric M. Gorman, Nashwa El-Gendy, Connor R. Bybee, Eric J. Munson, and Cory Berkland. 2009. "Nifedipine nanoparticle agglomeration as a dry powder aerosol formulation strategy." *International Journal of Pharmaceutics* 369 (1–2):136-143. doi: 10.1016/j.ijpharm.2008.10.016.

Prota, Lucia, Antonietta Santoro, Maurizio Bifulco, Rita P Aquino, Teresa Mencherini, and Paola Russo. 2011. "Leucine enhances aerosol performance of Naringin dry powder and its activity on cystic fibrosis airway epithelial cells." *International Journal of Pharmaceutics* 412 (1):8-19.

Rabbani, Naumana R., and Peter C. Seville. 2005. "The influence of formulation components on the aerosolisation properties of spray-dried powders." *Journal of Controlled Release* 110 (1):130-40. doi: 10.1016/j.jconrel.2005.09.004.

Rattanupatam, Teerarat, and Teerapol Srichana. 2014. "Budesonide dry powder for inhalation: Effects of leucine and mannitol on the efficiency of delivery." *Drug Delivery* 21 (6):397-405. doi: 10.3109/10717544.2013.868555.

Rawat, Amit, Quamrul H. Majumder, and Fakhrul Ahsan. 2008. "Inhalable large porous microspheres of low molecular weight heparin: In vitro and in vivo evaluation." *Journal of Controlled Release* 128 (3):224-232. doi: 10.1016/j.jconrel.2008.03.013.

Rojanarat, Wipaporn, Narumon Changsan, Ekawat Tawithong, Sirirat Pinsuwan, Hak-Kim Chan, and Teerapol Srichana. 2011. "Isoniazid proliposome powders for inhalation-preparation, characterization and cell culture studies." *International Journal of Molecular Sciences* 12 (7):4414-4434. doi: 10.3390/ijms12074414.

Rojanarat, Wipaporn, Titpawan Nakpheng, Ekawat Thawithong, Niracha Yanyium, and Teerapol Srichana. 2012a. "Inhaled pyrazinamide proliposome for targeting alveolar macrophages." *Drug Delivery* 19 (7):334-345. doi: 10.3109/10717544.2012.721144.

Rojanarat, Wipaporn, Titpawan Nakpheng, Ekawat Thawithong, Niracha Yanyium, and Teerapol Srichana. 2012b. "Levofloxacin-proliposomes: opportunities for use in lung tuberculosis." *Pharmaceutics* 4 (3):385-412.

Seville, Peter C., Tristan P. Learoyd, Haoying Li, Ian J. Williamson, and James C. Birchall. 2007. "Amino acid-modified spray-dried powders with enhanced aerosolisation properties for pulmonary drug delivery." *Powder Technology* 178 (1):40-50. doi: 10.1016/j.powtec.2007.03.046.

Sivadas, Neeraj, Desmond O'Rourke, Aoife Tobin, Vivienne Buckley, Zeibun Ramtoola, John G Kelly, Anthony J Hickey, and Sally-Ann Cryan. 2008. "A comparative study of a range of polymeric microspheres as potential carriers for the inhalation of proteins." *International Journal of Pharmaceutics* 358 (1):159-167.

Smith, Dan J., Linda M. Gambone, Thomas Tarara, Diana R. Meays, Luis A. Dellamary, Catherine M. Woods, and Jeffry Weers. 2001. "Liquid dose pulmonary instillation of gentamicin PulmoSpheres® formulations: Tissue distribution and pharmacokinetics in rabbits." *Pharmaceutical Research* 18 (11):1556-1561. doi: 10.1023/a:1013078330485.

Srichana, Teerapol, Roongnapa Suedee, and Wantana Reanmongkol. 2001. "Cyclodextrin as a potential drug carrier in salbutamol dry powder aerosols: The in-vitro deposition and toxicity studies of the complexes." *Respiratory Medicine* 95 (6):513-519. doi: 10.1053/rmed.2001.1079.

Steckel, Hartwig, and Nina Bolzen. 2004. "Alternative sugars as potential carriers for dry powder inhalations." *International Journal of Pharmaceutics* 270 (1):297-306.

Steckel, Hartwig, and Heike G. Brandes. 2004. "A novel spray-drying technique to produce low density particles for pulmonary delivery." *International Journal of Pharmaceutics* 278 (1):187-195. doi: 10.1016/j.ijpharm.2004.03.010.

Tang, Patricia, Hak-Kim Chan, Herbert Chiou, Keiko Ogawa, Matthew D. Jones, Handoko Adi, Graham Buckton, Robert K. Prud'homme, and Judy Agnes Raper. 2009. "Characterisation and aerosolisation of mannitol particles produced via confined liquid impinging jets." *International Journal of Pharmaceutics* 367:51-57.

Tarara, Thomas E, Michael S Hartman, Howard Gill, Alan A Kennedy, and Jeffry G Weers. 2004. "Characterization of suspension-based metered dose inhaler formulations composed of spray-dried budesonide microcrystals dispersed in HFA-134a." *Pharmaceutical Research* 21 (9):1607-1614.

Telko, Martin J, and Anthony J Hickey. 2005. "Dry powder inhaler formulation." *Respiratory Care* 50 (9):1209-1227.

Tewes, Frederic, Carsten Ehrhardt, and Anne Marie Healy. 2014. "Superparamagnetic iron oxide nanoparticles (SPIONs)-loaded Trojan microparticles for targeted aerosol delivery to the lung." *European Journal of Pharmaceutics and Biopharmaceutics* 86 (1):98-104. doi: 10.1016/j.ejpb.2013.09.004.

Tsapis, Nicolas, David Bennett, Blair Jackson, David A Weitz, and DA Edwards. 2002. "Trojan particles: large porous carriers of nanoparticles for drug delivery." *Proceedings of the National Academy of Sciences* 99 (19):12001-12005.

Ungaro, Francesca, Giuseppe De Rosa, Agnese Miro, Fabiana Quaglia, and Maria Immacolata La Rotonda. 2006. "Cyclodextrins in the production of large porous particles: Development of dry powders for the sustained release of insulin to the lungs." *European Journal of Pharmaceutical Sciences* 28 (5):423-432. doi: 10.1016/j.ejps.2006.05.005.

Ungaro, Francesca, Concetta Giovino, Ciro Coletta, Raffaella Sorrentino, Agnese Miro, and Fabiana Quaglia. 2010. "Engineering gas-foamed large porous particles for efficient local delivery of macromolecules to the lung." *European Journal of Pharmaceutical Sciences* 41 (1):60-70. doi: 10.1016/j.ejps.2010.05.011.

Upadhyay, Dhrumil, Santo Scalia, Robert Vogel, Nial Wheate, Rania O Salama, Paul M Young, Daniela Traini, and Wojciech Chrzanowski. 2012. "Magnetised thermo responsive lipid vehicles for targeted and controlled lung drug delivery." *Pharmaceutical Research* 29 (9):2456-2467.

Vemuri, Sriram, and Christopher T. Rhodes. 1995. "Preparation and characterization of liposomes as therapeutic delivery systems: a review." *Pharmaceutica Acta Helvetiae* 70 (2):95-111.

Weers, Jeffry G, Andrew R Clark, Nagaraja Rao, Keith Ung, Alfred Haynes, Sanjeev K Khindri, Sheryl A Perry, Surendra Machineni, and Paul Colthorpe. 2015. "In vitro–in vivo correlations observed with indacaterol-based formulations delivered with the breezhaler®." *Journal of Aerosol Medicine and Pulmonary Drug Delivery* 28 (4):268-280.

Wong, William, David F. Fletcher, Daniela Traini, Hak-Kim Chan, John Crapper, and Paul M. Young. 2010. "Particle aerosolisation and break-up in dry powder inhalers 1: Evaluation and modelling of venturi effects for agglomerated systems." *Pharmaceutical Research* 27 (7):1367-1376. doi: 10.1007/s11095-010-0128-4.

Xu, Zhen, Heidi M Mansour, Tako Mulder, Richard Mclean, John R. Langridge, and Anthony J Hickey. 2010. "Dry powder aerosols generated by standardized entrainment tubes from drug blends with lactose monohydrate: 1. Albuterol sulfate and disodium cromoglycate." *Journal of Pharmaceutical Sciences* 99 (8):3398-3414. doi: 10.1002/jps.22107.

Yang, Yan, Nimisha Bajaj, Peisheng Xu, Kimberly Ohn, Michael D. Tsifansky, and Yoon Yeo. 2009. "Development of highly porous large PLGA microparticles for pulmonary drug delivery." *Biomaterials* 30 (10):1947-1953. doi: 10.1016/j.biomaterials.2008.12.044.

Chapter 6

Device Design and Delivery Efficiency

6.1. Introduction

Asthma is one example of a respiratory disease where airways develop hyperresponsiveness and inflammation occur. Inhalation of drugs has been targeted primarily to inhibit both the release of mediators (e.g., sodium cromoglycate) and their action (e.g., a histamine/amine derivative antagonist), and to treat the results of mediator action (e.g., β_2 agonists, corticosteroids). Other uses of aerosol therapy include the use of mucolytics that will control abnormal mucus secretions and antibiotics for lung infections. Aerosol technology has been used productively for the treatment of respiratory diseases and when the prime requirement of that aerosol particle is to deposit the drug in the lung.

There are several factors that can affect the deposition of pharmaceutical aerosols in the lung as mentioned in the earlier chapter but all still pertain to the patient, the delivery device or the formulation. Any proposed delivery system should provide a high drug deposition both *in vitro* and *in vivo*.

The particle size has a major role in determining the site and amount of drug deposited within the respiratory system. To date, inhalation delivery has been based around three broad delivery systems: metered dose inhalers; nebulizers and DPIs. These three inhaler systems that are capable of dispensing such particles will be considered in terms of their different delivery mechanisms.

6.2. Classifications of
Dry Powder Inhalers

DPIs can be categorized into three types based on their design. The first group is comprised of single unit dose systems (usually employing a capsule) that include Spinhaler®, Rotahaler®, Inhalator® and Cyclohaler® devices. The second type employs multiple unit dose dispensing systems and examples are the Diskhaler® and Accuhaler®. The third class of DPI is a group of devices that contain multiple doses such as the Turbuhaler®, Autohaler®, Easyhaler® and Chiesi®. In a DPI, the drug is placed between the inlet and outlet of a passage through which air is inspired by the patient. Difficulties can arise in producing sufficient air flow through the device to entrain the drug and carry it as far as possible into the patient's lung. Air turbulence generated through the device and oral cavity dictates, in part, the amount of drug reaching the lower airways. The use of a capsule as a unit container such as the Spinhaler®, Rotahaler®, Inhalator® and Cyclohaler® is convenient and often does not lead to a marked loss of the drug through residual formulations that remain in the container after activation. However, moisture retention by the gelatin capsule and drug might cause problems with the stability of the drug and the ease of powder dispersion.

Hence, a subsequent generation of multiple unit dose devices has emerged to solve such problems by protecting the drug from moisture until the point of administration. However, in some of these newer devices, the FPF has not shown much improvement. The dose uniformity in some multiple dose systems can be poor. Multiple dose inhalers may, therefore, require filling with more drug than is needed to maintain a dose uniformity until the last dose was dispensed.

6.3. Dry Powder Inhaler Device Resistances

The respiratory flow rate at which a patient inhales through a DPI device significantly affects the amount of drug reaching the lung. The energy produced by the inspiration disperses the drug powder exiting the device. The interaction between the device design, the pressure drop and the flow rates generated by the patient are the prime factors that affect not only the efficacy of the drug delivery but also influence the *in vitro* test. The internal resistance of the DPI device is measured using an in-house designed apparatus. The apparatus consists of a sealed metal box, approximately 1800 cm³, with a Perspex® cover housing the device. The device is held between two Teflon ring seals. One side of the box is connected to a pump. Air is drawn through the apparatus at various flow rates by adjusting an air flow rotameter. The experimental set up for a resistance measurement of a DPI is shown in Figure 6.1. The pressure drop across the apparatus containing the device is recorded by a digital manometer (Extech®, Waltham, MA, USA). The difference in the pressure drop is determined with and without the device in place, and this is defined as the specific pressure drop of that device at a particular flow rate. The device resistance is calculated using the pressure drop and the flow rate as shown in the equation. The square root of the pressure drop versus the flow rate on the X-axis is plotted; the slope of the graph is the specific resistance of the device (R_D) as shown in equation 6.1.

$$\sqrt{\Delta P_D} = R_D Q \qquad (6.1)$$

Where,

P_D = the pressure drop across the device (mbar)

R_D = the specific resistance of the device (mbar$^{1/2}$/LPM)

Q = flow rate (LPM)

The specific resistance of the device is related to the pressure drop across the device (Srichana, Martin, and Marriott 1998). A linear relationship has been shown to exist between the square root of the pressure drop versus the flow rate for six inhaler devices in human volunteers (Rotahaler®, Spinhaler®, Cyclohaler®, Diskhaler®, Turbuhaler® and Inhalator Ingelheim®) as shown by equation 6.1 (Srichana, Martin, and Marriott 1998). The lowest resistance device was found to be the Rotahaler® followed by the Spinhaler®, Cyclohaler®, Diskhaler®, Turbuhaler® and the Inhalator Ingelheim®, respectively.

Amongst inhalers, DPIs play a major role in aerosol delivery for humans. However, due to the complexity of the peripheral airways, lungs and the physical mechanisms that govern aerosol delivery, the development of this kind of device and associated powder formulations remains mainly empirical.

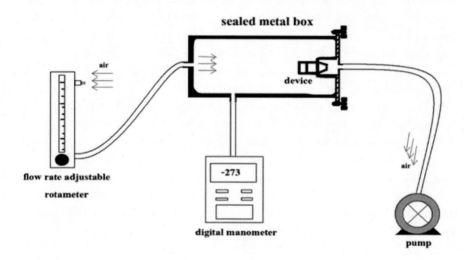

Figure 6.1. Device resistance measurement apparatus.

A measure of the aerosol delivery efficiency is often done in the laboratory by employing an apparatus specially designed for the aerodynamic assessment of fine particles by inertial impaction (e.g., the TSI or the ACI). In addition, it is assumed that the delivery efficiency is significantly determined by the FPF in the aerosol. This fraction shows the highest probability of depositing in the lower airways, a process that depends on numerous variables including the characteristics of the powder formulation and the specific features of the inhaler device.

The inhaler device produces a pressure drop as the air passes through it. The pressure drop is defined as the difference between the values of static pressure measured at two points in a system. A higher flow resistance leads to a larger pressure drop and ultimately produces a lower flow rate, for the same inhalation effort. However, a higher pressure drop in the device, that resulted from the narrow passage areas for the air flow, may also present a beneficial effect on the generation of fine particles (Srichana, Martin, and Marriott 1998). The larger shear stresses that act on the particles and/or the higher local turbulence lead to a better de-agglomeration of the powders. As a consequence, the inhalation of smaller-sized individual particles that are able to reach the lungs was promoted. The opposite effect was observed when the decrease in the inlet mouthpiece size resulted in an increased particle velocity release from the device. This caused a drug loss via inertial impaction (Figure 6.2) (DeHaan and Finlay 2004).

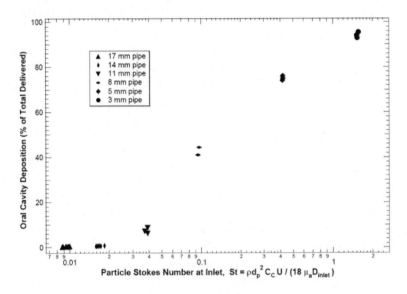

Figure 6.2. Oral cavity deposition for a 5 μm diameter aerosol at 32 LPM entering through various diameter straight tube inlets. (Reprinted from DeHaan, W. H. and Finlay, W. H., Journal of Aerosol Science, 35(3), 309-331, 2004. With permission from Elsevier).

Thus, a decrease of the diameter of the device inlet mouthpiece may be useful to produce a high turbulence air-flow through the device. However, it is necessary to be aware that it may cause a drug loss in the oral cavity via inertial impaction.

Olsson and Asking (1994a) have suggested using different flow rates to determine the dose emission from the devices *in vitro*. For example, 30 LPM was suggested to be most suitable for high resistance devices such as the Inhalator Ingelheim®, 60 LPM for the Turbuhaler® and 100-120 LPM for the

Spinhaler®, Rotahaler® and Diskhaler® (Hindle and Byron 1995). Brindley et al., (1994) characterized DPI devices using an inhalation simulator that generated typical *in vivo* conditions on the grounds that one constant flow rate could not predict the variation in clinical efficacy. This is because the inspiratory flow rate generated by an individual patient depends on the air flow resistance in different devices. The inhalation simulator was operated on the basis of a pressure drop rather than the flow rate and was designed to mimic the human inhalation profile of pressure drop versus time.

6.4. Dry Powder Inhaler Technology

The concept of the DPI technology is to transport a drug to the pulmonary system by use of the self-breathing of patients that aims to provide an accelerated release of the drug from the container and for the fine particles of the dry powder drug to reach the deep lung. This method was developed in 1967 to transport a sodium cromoglycate powder for the treatment of asthma.

The advantages of this technique are: use of a small amount of active compound; less systemic side effects compared to the oral route; an increase in the efficacy by avoiding first-pass metabolism in the liver; simple to operate when compared to the pMDI and no need for a propellant. Today this administration technique is admired in major targeted drug delivery systems for the treatment of pulmonary disease and plays a major role in a novel pathway for drug delivery.

Commonly, the degree of drug deposition performance depends on the forces of interaction within the powder formulation and the mechanical forces of dispersion from the device and the patient's inspiration effort (Louey, Razia, and Stewart 2003).

6.4.1. Device Factors

All DPIs have four basic features to release drug particles from the device: (1) a dose metering mechanism; (2) an aerosolization mechanism; (3) a deaggregation mechanism and (4) an adaptor to direct the aerosol into the patient's mouth. Drug particles are theoretically stripped from the surface of the lactose particles on which they are loosely attached during the generation process. This process is illustrated schematically in Figure 6.3. Thus, the drug particles are dispersed and can traverse the upper respiratory tract, while the excipient particles do not pass beyond the mouthpiece of the device or the mouth and throat of the patient (Tiano and Dalby 1996).

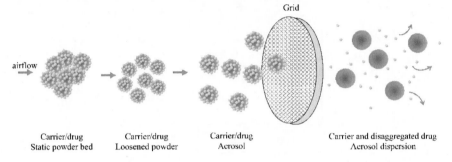

Figure 6.3. Mechanism of drug release from dry powder inhaler. (Redrawn from Tiano S. L. and Dalby, R. N., Pharmaceutical Development and Technology, 1(3), 261-268, 1996).

The design of the device is a crucial factor for the DPI delivery performance. In common, the device must be able to generate a force that results in the de-agglomeration of the particles to generate the fine drug particles (deaggregation mechanism). The concept on how the powder interacts with the device during dispersion is generally classified into 3 types of impaction. Air turbulence and mechanical impaction (particle–particle, particle–device surface) are generally accepted as mechanisms controlling powder dispersion in the device (Figure 6.4). As a result, fine drug particles are generated and are delivered to the deep lung.

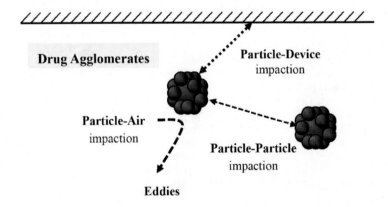

Figure 6.4. Mechanisms of dispersion of the powder as aerosol inside an inhaler.

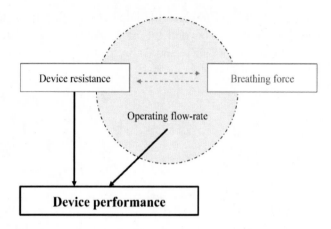

Figure 6.5. Relationship between the device resistance, the breathing force and the device performance.

An interesting impaction behavior that results from the device design is the device resistance (Figure 6.5). The device resistance is related to the breathing force. A high device resistance requires a higher effort from the patients that directly affects the operating flow rate. However, the high device resistance provides a high degree of turbulent air-flow inside the device, which in turn increases the performance of the device. In conclusion, the device should create a balance between the optimal resistance and the optimal turbulence of the air-flow (Srichana, Martin, and Marriott 1998).

Table 6.1. Characteristics required for an ideal dry powder inhaler (Ashurst et al. 2000)

Effective dosing	Efficient device	Easy to use
• Uniform dose throughout its life • Targeted and optimized delivery • Controlled respirable fraction • Inhalation of dose-independent aerosol generation • Bolus of aerosol available at the beginning of an inhalation • Operatable at low flow rates	• Good environmental protection • In-process controls for quality • Compact, portable, cheap and/or reusable • Clear comparative data for administration compliance	• Simple operation • Dose counter • Dose-ready indicator • Patient feedback of dose administration

For the present competition in the DPI market today, every company must improve their product design to gain customer satisfaction in addition to the performance of drug delivery. There are lists of possible requirements for an ideal DPI, which are summarized in Table 6.1.

6.4.2. Disposable Dry Powder Inhalers

Disposable DPIs provide the pulmonary drug delivery of single-dose applications (e.g., inhaled vaccination). The design of disposable DPIs is quite different from that of the multi-dose counterparts. In addition to the general requirements of dose uniformity and deposition, the disposable DPIs should have features of simple operation with low costs. The TwinCaps® is an example of a disposable DPI device for delivery of laninamivir octanoate (Inavir®), a long-acting neuraminidase inhibitor prodrug for the treatment of influenza. It is different from the short acting zanamivir that requires twice daily for five days. A single dose of 40 mg inhaled laninamivir can be effective for a week, making it a perfect candidate. The design of the TwinCaps® is simple, with only two assembled plastic parts. Since the Inavir® TwinCaps® has been approved for children less than 10 years old, an aerosolization performance at lower flow rates is necessary.

The Twincer™ is a disposable device used to deliver colistin for the treatment of cystic fibrosis (CF). It has three plastic parts that can be easily assembled by stacking and clicking three pieces together. The formulation is packed in a blister-like compartment. The powders are dispersed through a multiple air classifier. Unlike Inavir® that requires only a single administration, inhaled colistin therapy for CF patients needs to be administered twice daily for at least 28 days. The disposable design is able to reduce the potential risk of bacterial contamination.

Aespira's resQhaler™ is a recently developed disposable DPI based on the ActiveMesh™ technology. The doses of resQhaler™ are up to 3 mg, which may limit its use until further design improvements can accommodate more powder.

6.4.3. Multiple Dose Dry Powder Inhalers

In multiple dose DPIs, the powder formulation is prefilled in a capsule or cartridge, which is then loaded into the device. With the storage compartment being separated from the inhaler, multiple dose inhalers can come with small dimensions. Since the device can be used many times, the cost of medication per dose is significantly reduced. In some cases, more than one dosing unit can be given, making dosing more flexible. Multiple dose devices are currently employed for high dose antibiotics. Both the TOBI® Podhaler® (tobramycin) and Colobreathe Turbospin® (colistimethate sodium) are capsule-based multiple dose DPIs. Passive reloadable devices can achieve satisfactory aerosol performance with minimized flow rate dependence when the drug powders are properly engineered.

6.5. Present Design of Commercial Dry Powder Inhaler Devices

DPI devices can be classified into 3 types based on drug dosing (Table 6.2). The single unit dose and multiple unit dose devices are factory metered doses whereas the multidose is immediately metered after use. The advantages of the single unit dose device are that each unit dose has environmental protection by the in-process control during factory dispensing and all of the single unit dose devices or even some multiple unit dose devices can be reused. The disadvantage of the single unit dose device is that the patient either needs to carry a separate reservoir or the device is not portable. The multidose devices provide ease of operation and can be portable compared to the unit dose systems, but the devices cannot be cleaned and reused.

Commercial DPI devices have different structures and delivery mechanisms. The main objective of the design of the device is to optimize the device resistance so that patients can inspire while producing good turbulent air-flow inside the device. Some mechanisms of turbulent air-flow production are illustrated below.

6.5.1. Spinhaler®

The Spinhaler® works by inserting the capsule into an impeller in the body of the inhaler. The capsule is pierced by the device pins when the system is ready to use (Figure 6.6). The patient inhales through the mouthpiece. Sodium cromoglycate deposition has been studied following delivery of the drug by inhalation to volunteers using the Spinhaler®. There was a marked difference between-subject variability in the plasma concentrations of sodium cromoglycate achieved and in the areas under the plasma concentration-time curves of the drug (Auty et al. 1987). This reflected the variability between different subjects on the amount of the drug delivered to the respiratory tract. Most of this variability was due to differences in the inhalation technique, particularly with regard to the inspiratory flow rate achieved and the duration of breath-holding after inhalation.

Table 6.2. Currently marketed dry powder inhaler devices.
(Adapted from Lavorini, F. et al., Respiratory, 88(1), 3-15, 2014 and
Berkenfeld, K. et al., AAPS PharmSciTech, 16(3), 479-490, 2015)

Device name	Type	Formulation Storage	Company
Spinhaler®	Single dose	Capsule	Aventis
Rotahaler®	Single dose	Capsule	GSK
Cyclohaler®/Aerolizer®	Single dose	Capsule	Pharmachemie/ Novartis
Handihaler®	Single dose	Capsule	Boehringer-Ingelheim
Turbuhaler®	Multiple dose	Reservoir	Astra Zeneca
Diskhaler®	Multiple unit dose	Blister pack	GSK
Diskus®	Multiple unis dose	Blister strip	GSK
Aerohaler	Single dose	Capsule	Boehringer-Ingelheim
Easyhaler®	Multiple dose	Reservoir	Orion
Pulvinal®	Multiple dose	Reservoir	Chiesi
NEXThaler®	Multiple dose	Reservoir	Chiesi
Novolizer®	Multiple dose	Cartridge	MEDA
Turbospin®	Single dose	Capsule	PH&T
Jethaler®	Multiple dose	Ring tablet	Ratiopharm
Taifun	Multiple dose	Reservoir	LAB Pharma
Clickhaler®	Multiple dose	Reservoir	Recipharm
Flexhaler™	Multiple dose	Reservoir	Astra Zeneca
Twisthaler®	Multiple dose	Reservoir	Schering-Plough
Genuair®	Multiple dose	Reservoir	Almirall
Clickhaler®	Multiple dose	Reservoir	Innovate Biomed
Ellipta™	Multiple unit dose	Strip	GSK
Airmax	Multiple unit dose	Reservoir	Norton Healthcare

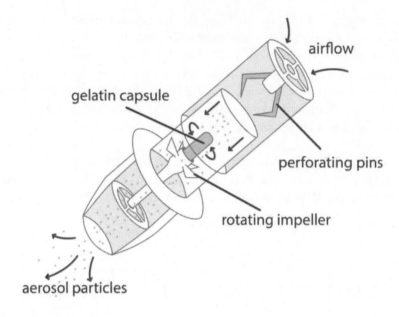

Figure 6.6. Spinhaler®.

6.5.2. Rotahaler®

The drug release from the Rotahaler® (GlaxoSmithKline, UK) is started by a separation of the body from the cap of the capsule. The release of the drug from the spinning capsule raises the particle impaction and passes through a crucial grating after the patient inhales through the Rotahaler® (Figure 6.7). The bronchodilator effects of the inhaled dry salbutamol powder (50, 100, 200 and 400 µg) have been compared in ten asthmatic patients with those of an aerosolized salbutamol (200 µg) delivered from a standard pressurized inhaler. The dose of the salbutamol powder (400 µg) produced a greater bronchodilation than the 50, 100 or 200 µg of powder, but there was no significant difference between the 400 µg of powder and the 200 µg of the aerosolized salbutamol (Hartley et al. 1977). Powder administered by the Rotahaler® was well tolerated and offered several advantages over the pressurized aerosol canister. Recently Sim et al. (2014) studied the powder fluidization and aerosolization processes in the Rotahaler®. The study focused on examining the effect of the different characteristics of the lactose carrier employed and specifically considered the powder fluidization, entrainment and

de-agglomeration mechanisms. The results showed that the powder fluidization from a dynamic split capsule was substantially different from those of a static powder bed. Furthermore, the presence of the split capsule dominated the powder emission mechanisms from the Rotahaler®, and this was regulated by its impaction on the grid/Rotahaler® wall and the rotational movement in the entrained air.

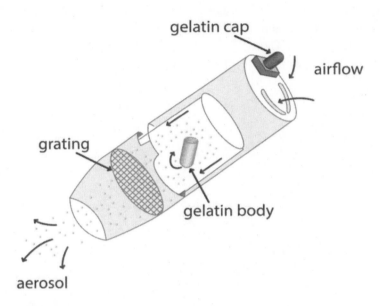

Figure 6.7. Rotahaler®.

6.5.3. Handihaler®

The Handihaler® works by inserting the capsule into the chamber and a button is then pressed to pierce the capsule. The patient then inhales the medication through the mouthpiece. The dry powder will be released from the pierced holes by the movement of the capsule like a piston. Many chronic obstructive pulmonary disease patients use their inhaler ineffectively. Inverse gas chromatography was used to assess the surface energy of the active (albuterol and ipratropium bromide) and carrier (lactose monohydrate, trehalose dihydrate, and mannitol) components of a DPI formulation. Blends (1%, w/w) of the drug and carrier were prepared and evaluated for the DPIs performance by cascade impaction. The formulations were tested with either of two passive DPIs, the Rotahaler® (GlaxoSmithKline) or the Handihaler®

(Boehringer Ingelheim). The *in vitro* performance of the powder blends was strongly correlated to the surface energy interactions between the active and carrier components (Cline and Dalby 2002). Increasing the surface energy interaction between the drug and carrier resulted in a greater FPF of the drug. One study compared the preference and the ease of use between Diskus® and Handihaler® (Van Der Palen et al. 2007). Patients had to state a preference for Diskus® or Handihaler®. Subsequently, they inhaled through a range of resistances and scored the acceptability. More patients preferred the Diskus® than the Handihaler®. There was no difference in the number of instructions needed for both inhalers to obtain a perfect inhalation technique.

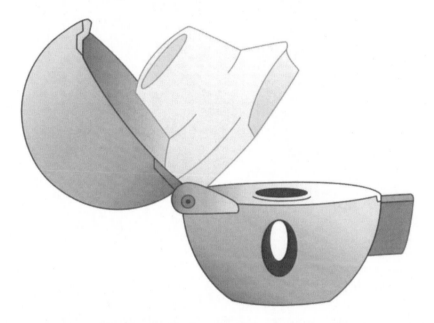

Figure 6.8. Handihaler (Redrawn from www.rpc-bramlage.de/Healthcare-en-01.html).

6.5.4. Diskhaler®

A Diskhaler® is a dry-powder inhaler that holds small blisters, each containing a dose of medication on a disk. The Diskhaler® punctures each blister so that its medication can be inhaled. An open, randomized, cross-over study was performed to compare the efficacy and acceptability of two breath-actuated inhalers, the Turbohaler® and the Diskhaler® for delivery of beta-agonists (Brown et al. 1992). Thirty-six adults with chronic asthma requiring beta-agonists four times daily were treated with terbutaline 500 μg via the Turbohaler® and salbutamol 400 μg via the Diskhaler® four times daily for four weeks. The peak expiratory flow (PEF) was recorded in the morning (before and after the beta-agonist) and the evening. The mean morning PEF was higher during the first two weeks of using the Turbohaler® (295 LPM) than the Diskhaler® (281 LPM), but this difference did not persist during the next two weeks and there were no differences in the post-bronchodilator PEF or use of the beta-agonist rescue. After four weeks, >90% of the patients used both inhaler devices efficiently and they were equally acceptable in terms of ease of use and convenience to carry. The Diskhaler® and Turbohaler® achieved similar clinical efficacy for the delivery of the beta-agonists.

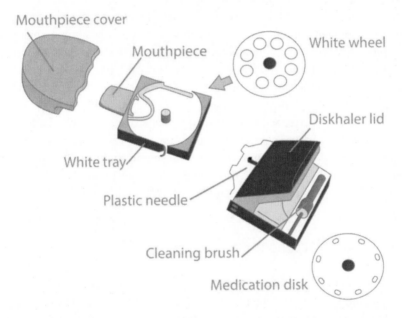

Figure 6.9. Diskhaler® (Redrawn from www.asthma.ca/adults/treatment/diskhaler.php).

6.5.5. Turbuhaler®

The Tubuhaler® is a cylindrical, multi-dose DPI device. The dosing is achieved by twisting the turning grip back and forth followed by deep inhalation. It contains 200 metered doses and is equipped with a dosage indicator window. The most interesting feature is the number of spiral channels in the device that can produce good fine particles of the drug even in the presence of drug-drug aggregate formulations (Figure 6.10). The Turbuhaler® is manufactured by AstraZeneca. It was one of the first DPIs to dispense metered doses from a reservoir inside the inhaler. The device is made up of plastic components and a steel spring, with a reservoir. It contains 50, 100 or 200 doses. Each dose is metered accurately regardless of the remaining dose. It is impossible for the patient to inhale an overdose. The patient will notice from the dose indicator when there are 20 doses or fewer remaining. When the grip at the base is fully twisted in one direction and back again a single dose is loaded. This action fills powder into conical holes in a rotating dosing disc, and scrapers then remove any surplus drug to ensure accurate dosing. Inhalation through the mouthpiece forces air through the holes in the dosing disc which transfers the powder into the deaggregation zone. This action occurs in the mouthpieces which are designed to create a turbulent flow. As the drug deaggregation is airflow dependent, extra air is admitted below the mouthpiece to reduce the pressure drop. The device presents an airflow resistance of 0.11 $(cmH_2O)^{1/2}/LPM$. The Turbohaler® has a protective cover which contains a desiccant to keep low moisture content in the reservoir for at least 200 open/close cycles. The loaded drug without carrier comprises soft aggregates of the micronized drug formed by spheronization. The Turbuhaler® emits a dose that is dependent on the inspiratory flow rate (moderate to high). The Turbuhaler® has been approved for budesonide (Pulmicort®, Spirocort®), formoterol (Oxis®), terbutaline (Aerodura®, Bricanyl®) and a combination of budesonide and formoterol (Symbicort®).

6.5.6. Diskus®/Accuhaler®

The patient operates the inhaler by sliding a lever that moves the next dose-containing a blister into place. A ratchet within the inhaler causes the device to click when the next dose is properly positioned. Priming the device in this way simultaneously peels the two layers of foil apart exposing the dose ready for inhalation. The Diskus® also incorporates a dose counter, which enables the patient to monitor the number of doses remaining in the device, and also has an integral outer case that serves to keep the device dust free and also resets the lever ready for the next dose. The Diskus® was designed to be simple to operate and contains a dose counter. The performance of the Diskus® has been compared with that of a well-established reservoir powder inhaler (Fuller 1995). The pharmaceutical assessment of the Diskus® has shown that

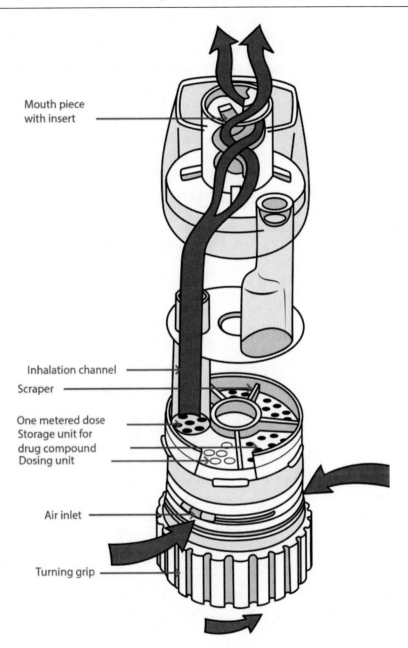

Figure 6.10. Turbuhaler® (Redrawn from
www.asthma.ca/images/adults/treatment/turbuhaler.gif).

the delivered dose of salmeterol and fluticasone propionate remains at approximately 90% of the labeled claim at flow rates of 30-90 LPM. This contrasts with data for the reservoir powder inhaler which showed that the delivered dose was lower than the labeled claim and more variable, particularly at flow rates of 30-60 LPM. The delivered dose from the Diskus® remains constant at different flow rates, unlike the reservoir powder inhaler, in which the fine particle mass is more dependent on the flow rate. The doses of the drug in the Diskus™ are protected from moisture. The FPF of salmeterol delivered from the Diskus® was unaffected by humidity (30°C/75% RH) as opposed to the reservoir powder inhaler in which the ingress of moisture was associated with a decrease in FPF. In clinical studies, salmeterol 50 µg twice daily and fluticasone propionate 50-500µg twice daily have been shown to be equally effective and well tolerated when delivered by Diskus® as compared with the Diskhaler®.

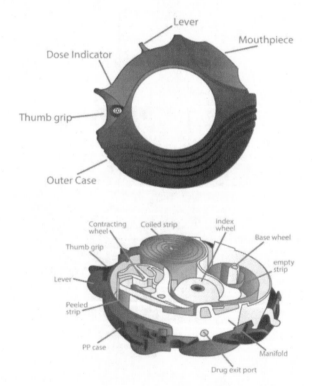

Figure 6.11. Diskus® inhaler (Redrawn from http://productdesignhub.com/2009/04/every-breath-you-take-dissecting-the-diskus/).

6.5.7. Easyhaler®

This powder device includes seven plastic parts. The powder is packaged into a powder reservoir from which the drug dose can be accurately measured by rotating the metering cylinder. This is realized by pushing down on the overcap of the device. The metered drug dose can then be inhaled through the mouthpiece which has been designed to redisperse the micronized drug particles from the surface of the carrier material. Thus the powder inhaler is constructed in such a way that its mode of use is similar to that of the MDI. The construction of the Easyhaler® allows high dose reproducibility and a good *in vitro* and *in vivo* deposition of the inhaled drug particles. In clinical studies with an equal therapeutic efficacy, the safety and tolerability to the MDI have been documented when salbutamol or beclomethasone dipropionate was delivered from an Easyhaler® to asthmatic adults or children. The FPF obtained from the Easyhaler® DPI remained relatively constant over the range of inspiratory flow rates from 30–60 LPM (Koskela et al. 2000).

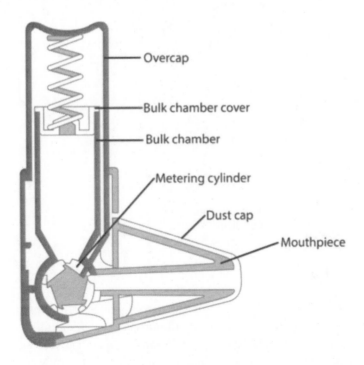

Figure 6.12. Easyhaler® (Redrawn from Clin Drug Invest © 2002 Adis International Limited).

6.5.8. NEXThaler®

This device comprises functional groups of components coupled together. The dosing mechanisms meter the drug from a reservoir, and the counting mechanisms include the breath-actuated mechanism that activates the dosing group under a certain air flow allowing the dose to be taken, and the dose counter to decrement only after an effective release of the therapeutic dose. There is a reservoir inside the device that houses the drug and every time a patient opens the cover and breathes through it, the right dose of the powder formulation is dispensed. To sense the user's breath, the device is equipped with a small vane that moves when the patient breathes and this triggers the dispensing mechanisms. Nexthaler® has a unique feedback system; a click is heard as a consequence of the activation of the breath-actuated mechanism and the dose counter decrements by one count only after the effective release of the dose.

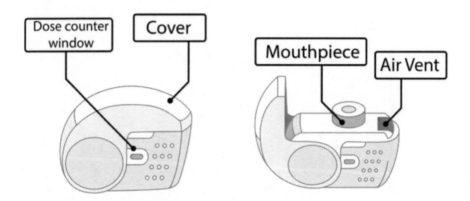

Figure 6.13. NEXThaler® (Redrawn from www.medicines.org.uk/emc/medicine/31250).

6.5.9. Exubera®

An insulin powder inhaler was developed by Nektar Therapeutics as Exubera® (Figure 6.14). A spray dried insulin powder is in unit dose blisters and a reusable inhaler. The device contains an air pump and valves, small jets (TransJector) and a mouthpiece. The inspiratory effort is power driven to deliver small amounts of cohesive powder (1–10 mg). A sonic discharge of air from the base through the TransJector upon actuation into the chamber de-agglomerates and disperses the inhalable powder into respirable aerosols. A clear holding chamber allows the patient to visualize the powder dispersal.

Exubera® was approved by the American and European Drug Agencies in 2006. However, Pfizer announced Exubera's removal from the market due to a failure to gain market acceptance in 2007.

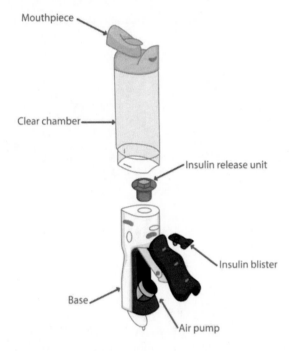

Figure 6.14. Exubera® (Redrawn from www.drugs.com/pro/exubera.html).

6.5.10. Podhaler™

The Podhaler™ (Novartis) is a portable, capsule-based, single-dose and multi-use DPI (Figure 6.15). A drug-containing capsule is loaded into the device by removing the mouthpiece and inserting the capsule into the chamber. The mouthpiece is screwed back onto the body. When the button is depressed to pierce the capsule, the patient inhales the DPI through the mouthpiece. During inspiration, the capsule rotates rapidly in the chamber which causes capsule emptying drug.

The Podhaler™ has a low airflow resistance of 0.08 $(cmH_2O)^{1/2}$/LPM to produce reliable dose delivery. A patient can empty a capsule with a 30-40

LPM flow rate and this result is an emitted dose of 90%. The Podhaler™ is marketed as the TOBI® tobramycin formulation using the PulmoSphere® technology. It is indicated for *Pseudomonas aeruginosa* infections in cystic fibrosis patients.

More recently, Bayer has launched phase III clinical trials of a ciprofloxacin DPI Respire® using the PulmoSphere® technology and a Podhaler™ for non-cystic fibrosis bronchiectasis patients.

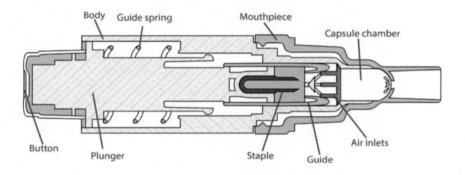

Figure 6.15. Redrawn Podhaler™ (Redrawn from Maltz, DS., and Paboojian, SJ., Proceedings of RDD Europe, 55-56, 2011).

6.5.11. Turbospin™

The Turbospin™ is a single-dose, multiuse DPI designed by PH&T for effective lung delivery. Its shape resembles a pen composed of a cap and a device for inhalation. The make-up of the plastic device consists of a mouthpiece and body. The body encloses the pulverization chamber and the piercing apparatus. The capsule is vertically inserted into the chamber and pierced by the needles at the bottom. Air is drawn through the designed chamber slits during inspiration which creates turbulence to empty the capsule. The drug in dry powder form is protected from moisture by packaging the capsule in the blister.

Turbospin is marketed as Colobreathe® by Forest Laboratories UK Ltd., which contains excipient-free micronized colistimethate sodium. It is active against *P. aeruginosa* that is commonly found in cystic fibrosis (Schuster et al. 2013).

6.5.12. Staccato®

Staccato® is a single-use inhaler designed by Alexza Pharmaceuticals which is based on powder sublimation (Figure 6.16). This is obtained by rapidly heating a thin film of the drug. The heating process is very quick in order to prevent thermal decomposition of the drug. It is triggered by the patient's inhalation, after sublimation the drug cools rapidly in the air and condenses into 1 to 3 µm aerosol. The aerosol is drawn into the patient's mouth and subsequently into the lungs. The emitted dose is ~90% of the drug and is independent of the patient's breathing pattern. As the device presents a valve that controls the airflow, a patient simply places the device to his or her lips and takes a deep breath. The Staccato® is marketed as loxapine Adasuve™. In addition, the device has been studied for the delivery of fentanyl, zaleplon, alprazolam and prochlorperazine. A multiple dose Staccato® is also under development.

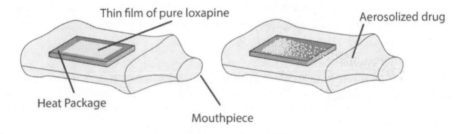

Thin film of pure loxapine

Aerosolized drug

Heat Package

Mouthpiece

Figure 6.16. Redrawn Staccato® (Redrawn from Dinh, K. et al., International Journal of Pharmaceutics, 403(1-2), 101-108, 2011).

6.6. Upcoming Devices

6.6.1. ARCUS® inhaler

The ARCUS® inhaler is a small, simple, portable, capsule-based, breath-actuated device that allows the delivery of single or multi-doses of a drug formulation using LPP technology. The device consists of two parts: a cylindrical chamber with multiple vents and a puncturing mechanism, and a second part consists of the mouthpiece and device body. Upon loading a capsule into the chamber, the puncturing mechanism creates two holes in the capsule. The powder is dispersed into the airways after inhalation. The device has a resistance of 0.28 (cm $H_2O)^{1/2}/$ LPM.

6.6.2. Cricket™ and Dreamboat™

MannKind Corporation has developed two devices: a single-use, disposable device called Cricket™ and a 15-day reusable device called Dreamboat™. The Dreamboat™ is currently used on dry powder insulin. The patient inhales the powder through the mouthpiece in a single breath. After the patient uses the device, the empty cartridge is removed and discarded.

The patient activates the Cricket™ by depressing the button and inhales the powder through the mouthpiece in a single breath.

Both devices present a common flow path: as a patient inhales, whereby two flow inlet streams converge simultaneously. The first inlet stream lifts the powder from a containment to deliver into a second by-pass inlet stream (Figure 6.17). The intersection of these two inlet streams de-agglomerates the fluidized powder, which then travels into the mouth. The powder dispersion occurs rapidly in the patient's inhalation maneuver.

In addition, the inhalers utilize a design that enables low flow rate use, which in turn reduces powder deposition in the oral cavity and promotes a deep lung deposition.

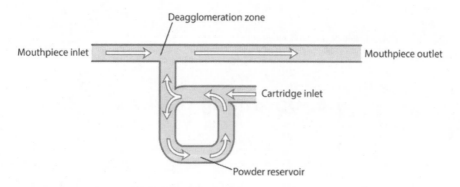

Figure 6.17. Design concept of Cricket™ and Dreamboat™ (Redrawn from Berkenfeld, K. et al., AAPS PharmSciTech, 16(3), 479-490, 2015).

6.6.3. 3M Taper™

The 3M Taper™ produced by the 3M Drug Delivery Systems is a multi-dose inhaler presenting the active drug on a microstructured carrier tape (MCT). The inhaler uses a "dimpled" tape to provide pre-metered doses. The dimple design allows for drug loading with the carrier; the loading is based on a balance between drug retention in the dimples and the drug release upon dosing. The cohesive drug is vital for this process. The drug delivered in each dose is determined by the number of dimples on the tape and by the volume of each dimple and the density of the drug packed into the dimples. Individual doses in the range of 100 µg to 1 mg are possible.

The device is compact and easy to use by only opening the device and a fixed length of the MCT is presented into the dosing zone. Upon inhaling, the air flow releases an impactor that strikes the tape and releases the drug into the airstream. The de-agglomeration of particles occurs as they pass through the device before closing. The device also provides a dose counter that is easy to read. The 3M Taper™ DPI is not currently in the market.

6.6.4. MicroDose

MicroDose Therapeutx, Inc., has developed an electronic DPI that utilizes a piezo vibrator to aerosolize the drug powders packaged in aluminum or plastic blisters (Figure 6.18). The device is designed for a single-dose or a multi-unit dose with disposable blisters.

It is operated in four steps: open cap; advance dose; inhale; close cap. Blisters are pierced with small needles prior to dosing into the flow channel of the device. Through breath activation, the piezo transducer converts electrical energy to vibration, creating an air pressure at the blister holes that levitate and disperse the powder. The powder emitted from the blister is aerosolized into the lungs. Because the piezo vibrator generates the energy for powder aerosolization, the dependent inspiratory flow is eliminated. The device is capable of delivering over 90% emitted dose, with the high fine particle fractions.

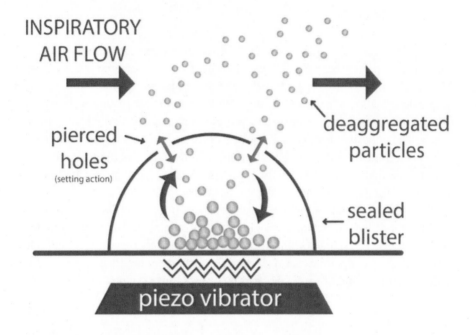

Figure 6.18. MicroDose DPI (Redrawn from Corcoran, T. E. et al., Journal of Aerosol Medicine and Pulmonary Drug Delivery, 26(1), 46-55, 2013).

6.6.5. Twincer™

The Twincer™ is a disposable DPI developed at the University of Groningen in the Netherlands (Figure 6.19). It is composed of three plate-like parts which constitute the air flow passages and a blister chamber containing the drug to be delivered. The blister has a long cover foil which connects the powder channel and the inlet to the blister chamber. Air passing through the powder channel during inhalation aerosolizes the powder from the blister. This powder flow is divided between two parallel classifiers. The inertial and shear forces act on the drug agglomerates resulting in de-agglomeration.

The device was designed for colistin and has been used for pulmonary delivery of peptides, proteins and vaccines. It was manufactured by Indes, (Netherlands) for clinical trials in cystic fibrosis. The University of Groningen continues their research on optimizing the Twincer™ for use in different formulations.

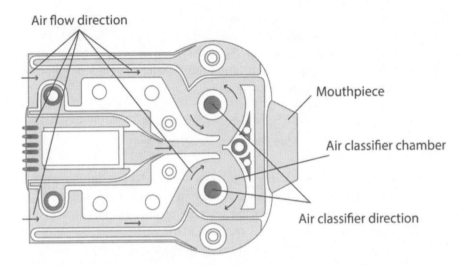

Figure 6.19. Twincer™ (Redrawn from Friebel, C. and Steckel, H., Expert Opinion on Drug Delivery, 7(12), 1359-1372, 2010).

6.6.6. Dry Powder Inhaler - The University of Western Ontario

The University of Ontario has developed a multi-dose DPI to deliver very small doses of drug to the lungs (100 - 500 µg). The powder is pre-metered in small pockets by a rotating multi-dose disc. The holes drilled the disc are placed between the air tubule and the compressing chamber in the air passage for a given dose. The double air flow design is applied to produce complete dispersion of the drug with the break-up of most agglomerates. After one dose is delivered, the disc can be rotated to set the next dose in the air passage. The emitted dose from the inhaler was found to vary between 88-92% with corresponding FPFs of 65- 69%.

6.7. Innovation in Dry Powder Inhaler Devices

The fine drug particles delivered to the lungs is determined by the balance of interparticulate forces within the powders, dispersion forces by airflow and deposition in the airways. Fine powders generated from micronization have high surface energy and cohesiveness. An inhaler device is necessary to disperse such powders into inhalable aerosols. The aerosolization behavior of a DPI depends on powder formulations and inhaler devices. While much effort has focused on the formulations in the past, there is a growing need to understand the device design. Innovation on inhaler design can provide improvements for powder aerosolization.

6.7.1. Design Modification for Passive Devices

The powder dispersion mechanisms in DPIs depend on the device resistance, air turbulence and impaction. Recent inhaler designs attempt to increase powder de-agglomeration by increasing the air turbulence and particulate collisions. The addition of collision in the airflow path can improve de-agglomeration. Such collision could be in the form of a 3D array of rods or an oscillating bead. However, not all the designs can substantially improve the aerosolization efficiency. For the Clickhaler®, the grid mesh does not increase the respirable doses of salbutamol sulfate or beclometasone dipropionate. The modifying grid affects not only the turbulence, but also the flow trajectory. In contrast, a modified Handihaler® equipped with a 3D array of rods in the mouthpiece improved the FPF from 87.6 to 97.3% of the emitted dose at 45 LPM. Computational fluid dynamics (CFD) analysis revealed that a much higher specific dissipation factor contributed to the improved aerosolization behavior compared to an unmodified device. Conix™ is a passive DPI device that utilized a reverse-flow cyclone technology to generate a high-velocity vortex to provide collision for de-agglomerated powders.

Other innovative design concepts go beyond the conventional approaches of generating shear forces and impactions by inhalation to disperse the powder. In a prototype device, an aero-elastic film coated with drug particles is fluttered by the inspiratory flow during operation. For high dose drugs, it is crucial to ensure sufficient loading on the film and consistent detachment of the particles from the film. A single-use DPI based on the ActiveMesh™ technology was developed with a mesh-sieving dispersion principle. The powder formulation was packed into a mesh inside the inhaler. The mesh package vibrates and forces the powder agglomerates to pass through the mesh holes to promote de-agglomeration during inhalation. Since the mesh vibration is a function of the airflow rate, device emptying and de-agglomeration may be a concern at low flow rates for cohesive powders. A 45 μm size mesh plus a turbulence-generation insert were shown to significantly improve the performance of the device (Zhou et al. 2014). In both fluttering and mesh-sieving designs, the airflow is not the direct source for powder dispersion. The de-agglomeration processes are still driven by the airflow rate.

6.7.2. Active Devices

Passive devices have been widely used for aerosolizing powder formulations. However, the dispersion performance of many devices suffers from being flow dependent. This problem is eliminated in the active devices that use external energy such as compressed air (e.g., Exubera® and Aspirair®), electrical vibration (e.g., MicroDose) and heat (e.g., Staccato®). However, active devices are not as popular as passive ones due to their high costs.

A multi-dose active device using compressed air has been recently developed to deliver micro-doses. Drug powders are pre-filled in small pocket holes drilled through a rotating disc, with only one drug pocket positioned in the air passage at a time. Two different compressed airflows are applied, where the primary flow disperses the drug powder from the pocket and the secondary flow fluidizes the powder into the primary flow. The FPF of spray dried insulin, phenylalanine, nitrendipine and phenylalanine ranged from 50 to 70%. This active device has the potential to deliver small amounts of cohesive powders which could be challenging.

A piezoelectric system has also been employed to aerosolize drug powders. Powders are stored in a blister in a MicroDose. When the inhaler is activated by inspiration, the blister is opened and the powders come in contact with a piezo vibrator. An atropine sulfate powder formulation aerosolized via the MicroDose DPI showed a FPF of 57% at a flow rate of 28.3 LPM. In Staccato®, drugs are coated onto a metallic strip and vaporized with a high temperature within 0.2 s. The drug vapor condenses and generates solid aerosols. The emitted doses were above 89% and the FPFs were 80–93% at flow rates of 15-45 LPM. It is worth noting that although the dispersion energy of the active devices does not rely on the inspiration flow, the oral deposition of aerosols is dependent on the patient's inhalation pattern. Thus, drug deposition in the oropharynx may vary substantially for patients with different inhalation capacities.

6.7.3. Future Directions in Dry Powder Inhaler Design

Passive devices based on traditional dispersion mechanisms will continue to dominate the DPI markets in the near future. In past decades, device efficiency was less significant as the majority of medications only required microgram drug doses.

However, this has become a crucial aspect with the increased interest of delivering high drug doses (>100 mg). It is challenging to deliver large amounts of powder without compromising the device portability and patient adherence. Furthermore, deposition of a high-dose powder in the oral cavity by a low-efficiency device could cause severe side effects such as coughing or irritation which results in the withdrawal of inhalation therapy. Most passive DPIs are only prescribed to patients aged > 6 years, leaving nebulisation to be the only choice for the younger children. Active DPIs can open a new window for the inhaled pediatric therapies. Another opportunity for active DPIs is in the critically ill patients. In the past, DPIs were unsuitable for patients who could not generate the required airflow to disperse the powder. Tang et al. (2011) have developed a novel powder delivery system that is suitable for patients with the aid of ventilation.

6.7.4. Computational Modeling

With the rapid advancements of the computational technologies, CFD has become a useful tool in providing information on flow patterns, turbulence levels and particle trajectories within the devices (Wong et al. 2012, Suwandecha, Wongpoowarak, and Srichana 2016). For the different approaches used for the dispersion of pharmaceutical aerosols, the corresponding advantages and limitations were reviewed by Wong et al. (2012) and Ruzycki et al. (2013). CFD modeling has been most prevalent for DPIs. However, the complicated processes involved in DPI dispersion have challenges to elucidate the underlying powder de-agglomeration mechanisms by pure numerical analysis. Therefore, a combination of CFD simulations and *in vitro* experiments is now commonly used to provide insights into the relative contributions of the various dispersion mechanisms (Figure 6.20) on the aerosolization performance (Suwandecha et al. 2016).

Coates et al. (2005, 2007) were among the first to use coupled CFD to study the Aerolizer® for a carrier-free formulation. The effects of the grid design, air inlet dimensions, capsule size, mouthpiece dimensions and air flow have been reported by Wong et al. (2012) and de Boer et al. (2012). Jiang et al. (2012) investigated further the effect of the height of the swirling chamber of the Aerolizer® and found improved aerosolization performance that was attributed to a lengthened powder–air interaction time. The performance of the Aerolizer® and HandiHaler® for carrier based formulations was investigated by Donovan et al. (2012). CFD analysis showed that the frequency of the carrier particle–inhaler collisions increased as the carrier particle size increased in the Aerolizer®, but not in the HandiHaler®. Therefore, they attributed this result to the improved aerosol performance of the larger lactose carrier formulations in the Aerolizer® to the higher carrier–inhaler collisions and suggested that impaction was the major de-agglomeration mechanism.

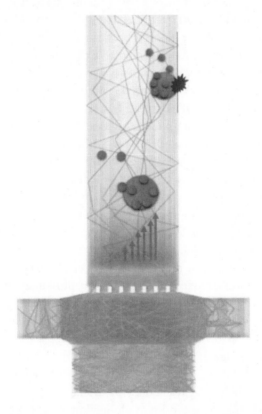

Figure 6.20. Particle dispersion mechanism in the cyclohaler. (Reprinted from Suwandecha, T. et al., Powder Technology, 267, 381-391, 2014. With permission from Elsevier).

Shur et al. (2012) also studied the flow characteristics within the HandiHaler® and Aerolizer® to identify the key features of the inhalers. They fabricated two modified versions of the Aerolizer® with the same specific resistances as the HandiHaler® to match the aerosol performance for the carrier-based Spiriva® formulation. These two modified designs exhibited very different cyclonic flows and only the one with similar flow properties to that of the HandiHaler® attained a comparable performance. Son, Y. et al. (2012) later utilized CFD to investigate the mouthpiece designs of the HandiHaler®.

With increased interest in developing high-dose DPIs, de Boer et al. (2012) evaluated computationally and experimentally the performance of the high-dose disposable Twincer™ to improve the product performance. The CFD results showed that the flow split was independent of the pressure drop across the inhaler and the bypass channel had little contribution to the swirl in the classifier. Therefore, they proposed blocking the bypass channel to reduce the total flow rate to minimize the mouth deposition without affecting the dispersion efficiency. To achieve quantitative analysis of the de-agglomeration mechanisms, specific interests have been placed to couple the CFD with the discrete element method (DEM) models that can take into account the mechanism of particle–particle, particle-fluid and particle–device interactions during powder dispersion. A coupled CFD-DEM approach was employed by Tong et al. (2010) to study the de-agglomeration of a single agglomerate comprising particles of various sizes and polydispersities in a cyclonic flow model similar to the Aerolizer®. They found that the breakup of the agglomerates into smaller fragments was governed by the particle–particle tensile strength and the particle–wall impact energy. Later, they used a two-way coupled CFD–DEM model to investigate the mechanism of powder de-agglomeration on mechanical impaction (Tong et al. 2011). They found that the first impaction only broke the agglomerate into small fragments with a weakened structure, while the subsequent impaction disintegrated them into fine particles. They further proposed that the FPF could be expressed as a unified error function of the ratio between the impaction energy and the strength of the agglomerate.

Tong et al. (2011) employed a fully coupled CFD–DEM model to study the dispersion of multiple agglomerates in the Aerolizer® and identified the particle–wall impaction as the primary de-agglomeration mechanism instead of the turbulence flow or particle–particle collisions. Sequential impactions of agglomerates with the inhaler base and grids led to a significant increase in the FPF. Though the dispersion mechanisms were elucidated, the information was specific for the formulation and device studied. Recently, CFD–DEM analysis coupled with *in vitro* experiments was applied to identify the critical features of the Aerolizer®. A CFD–DEM showed that the high-velocity particle–wall impactions in the inhaler dispersion chamber contributed mainly to the detachment of fine drug particles from the coarse carriers.

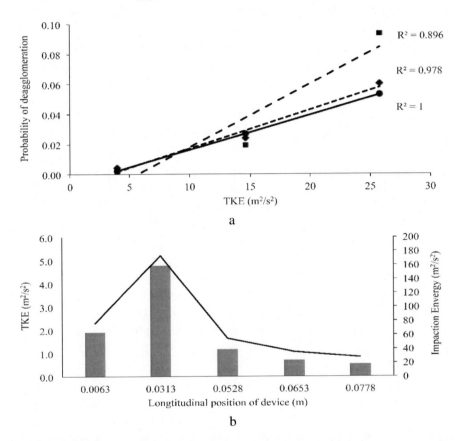

Figure 6.21. Correlation of TKE and probability of deagglomeration in Cyclohaler® device with fine (♦, dotted line), medium (■, dash line) and large (●, solid line) lactose carrier formulations (A), and TKE (bar) and impaction (line) energy along longitudinal length of the Cyclohaler® at 60 LPM using medium sized lactose carriers (B). (Reprinted from Suwandecha, T. et al., Powder Technology, 267, 381-391, 2014. With permission from Elsevier).

CFD–DEM modeling is time-consuming compared to the CFD alone. However, with the increase in the power of advanced processors, it is envisaged that advanced computations will play a more pivotal role in inhaler design in the near future.

Recently, Suwandecha et al. (2016) used a simpler computational method than the CFD-DEM by the CFD and discrete particle model. It was found that the particles de-agglomerated in two different ways: by aerodynamic shear dispersion and mechanical impaction de-agglomeration in that respective order. The aerodynamic shear force created stress on particle agglomeration and separated them. It was found that the turbulent kinetic energy (TKE) was a key parameter that described the aerodynamic shear force. If the TKE overcomes the interparticulate force, it will break the agglomerated particles (Figure 6.21).

6.7.5. Emerging Dry Powder Inhaler approaches

DPIs can be grouped into four categories: multi-unit, multi-dose reservoir, reusable single dose and single-use devices. The choice of the device is dependent on the dose, the dosing frequency and the powder properties. Multi-dose devices are popular for the frequently used medicines such as the anti-asthmatic drugs. There has been an increasing emphasis on simplifying the operation procedure to reduce incorrect device operation and improve patient adherence. For example, the NEXThaler® is a multi-dose inhaler designed with a simple operation procedure. A full dose feedback system was built into the NEXThaler® using a breath-actuated mechanism. The inhaler is activated only with a certain inspiratory flow to avoid miscounting if the dose is not inhaled. In a randomized cross-over study of the NEXThaler®, Diskus® and Turbuhaler® in 66 subjects, the NEXThaler® was rated as the easiest to use and the most preferred inhaler with a significantly lower number of usage errors (Voshaar et al. 2014). Reloadable or reusable inhalers were the most favorable to administer frequently used medications. Most capsule-based DPIs belong to this group and are still active in the DPI market. In the last five years, there has been an increasing trend to explore new applications of DPI to deliver antimicrobials, vaccines or other single-dose active ingredients. As such, single-use devices serve the purpose of that particular therapy.

References

Ashurst, Ian, Ann Malton, David Prime, and Barry Sumby. 2000. "Latest advances in the development of dry powder inhalers." *Pharmaceutical Science & Technology Today* 3 (7):246-256. doi: 10.1016/S1461-5347(00)00275-3.

Auty, Richard M, Kevan Brown, Michael G Neale, and Phillip D Snashall. 1987. "Respiratory tract deposition of sodium cromoglycate is highly dependent upon technique of inhalation using the Spinhaler." *British Journal of Diseases of the Chest* 81:371-380.

Berkenfeld, Kai, Alf Lamprecht, and Jason T. McConville. 2015. "Devices for Dry Powder Drug Delivery to the Lung." *AAPS PharmSciTech* 16 (3):479-490. doi: 10.1208/s12249-015-0317-x.

Brindley, Anne, Barry S Sumby, and Ian J Smith. 1994. "The characterisation of inhalation devices by an inhalation simulator: the Electronic Lung™." *Journal of Aerosol Medicine* 7 (2):197-200.

Brown, Peter H., Jill Lenney, Susan W. Armstrong, AC W S Ning, and Graham K Crompton. 1992. "Breath-actuated inhalers in chronic asthma: comparison of Diskhaler and Turbohaler for delivery of beta-agonists." *European Respiratory Journal* 5 (9):1143-1145.

Cline, David, and Richard Dalby. 2002. "Predicting the quality of powders for inhalation from surface energy and area." *Pharmaceutical Research* 19 (9):1274-1277.

Coates, Matthew S, Hak-Kim Chan, David F Fletcher, and Herbert Chiou. 2007. "Influence of mouthpiece geometry on the aerosol delivery performance of a dry powder inhaler." *Pharmaceutical Research* 24 (8):1450-1456.

Coates, Matthew S, Hak-Kim Chan, David F Fletcher, and Judy A Raper. 2005. "Influence of air flow on the performance of a dry powder inhaler using computational and experimental analyses." *Pharmaceutical Research* 22 (9):1445-1453.

Coates, Matthew S, David F Fletcher, Hak-Kim Chan, and Judy A Raper. 2005. "The role of capsule on the performance of a dry powder inhaler using computational and experimental analyses." *Pharmaceutical Research* 22 (6):923-932.

Corcoran, Timothy Edward, Raman V. Venkataramanan, Robert M. Hoffman, Meera Patricia George, Andrej A. Petrov, Thomas J. Richards, Shimin Zhang, Jiyeon Choi, Y. Y. Gao, C. D. Oakum, R. O. Cook, and Michael P. Donahoe. 2013. "Systemic Delivery of Atropine Sulfate by the MicroDose Dry-Powder Inhaler." *Journal of Aerosol Medicine and Pulmonary Drug Delivery* 26 (1):46-55. doi: 10.1089/jamp.2011.0948.

de Boer, Anne H, Paul Hagedoorn, Robert Woolhouse, and Ed Wynn. 2012. "Computational fluid dynamics (CFD) assisted performance evaluation of the Twincer™ disposable high-dose dry powder inhaler." *Journal of Pharmacy and Pharmacology* 64 (9):1316-1325.

DeHaan, Wesley H., and Warren H Finlay. 2004. "Predicting extrathoracic deposition from dry powder inhalers." *Journal of Aerosol Science* 35 (3):309-331.

Dinh, Khe, Dan J. Myers, Marc Glazer, Tamara Shmidt, Caitlin Devereaux, Kathleen Simis, Peter D. Noymer, Min He, Corinna Choosakul, Qiang Chen, and James V. Cassella. 2011. "In vitro aerosol characterization of Staccato® Loxapine." *International Journal of Pharmaceutics* 403 (1–2):101-108. doi: 10.1016/j.ijpharm.2010.10.030.

Donovan, Martin J, Sin HYEN Kim, Venkatramanan Raman, and Hugh D Smyth. 2012. "Dry powder inhaler device influence on carrier particle performance." *Journal of Pharmaceutical Sciences* 101 (3):1097-1107.

Friebel, Christian, and Hartwig Steckel. 2010. "Single-use disposable dry powder inhalers for pulmonary drug delivery." *Expert Opinion on Drug Delivery* 7 (12):1359-1372. doi: 10.1517/17425247.2010.538379.

Fuller, Rick. 1995. "The Diskus™: a new multi-dose powder device–efficacy and comparison with Turbuhaler™." *Journal of Aerosol Medicine* 8 (s2):S-11-S-17.

Hartley, Julie P. R., Stephan G. Nogrady, Owain M. Gibby, and Anthony W. H. Seaton. 1977. "Bronchodilator effects of dry salbutamol powder administered by Rotahaler." *British Journal of Clinical Pharmacology* 4 (6):673-675.

Hindle, Michael, and Peter R Byron. 1995. "Dose emissions from marketed dry powder inhalers." *International Journal of Pharmaceutics* 116 (2):169-177.

Jiang, Liqun, Yue Tang, Hongjiu Zhang, Xifeng Lu, Xijing Chen, and Jiabi Zhu. 2012. "Importance of powder residence time for the aerosol delivery performance of a commercial dry powder inhaler Aerolizer®." *Journal of Aerosol Medicine and Pulmonary Drug Delivery* 25 (5):265-279.

Koskela, Tommi, Kristiina Malmström, Ulla Sairanen, S Peltola, Juha Keski-Karhu, and Matti S L Silvasti. 2000. "Efficacy of salbutamol via Easyhaler® unaffected by low inspiratory flow." *Respiratory Medicine* 94 (12):1229-1233.

Lavorini, Federico, Giovanni Fontana, and Omar Sharif Usmani. 2014. "New Inhaler Devices - The Good, the Bad and the Ugly." *Respiration* 88 (1):3-15.

Louey, Margaret D., Sultana Razia, and Peter J. Stewart. 2003. "Influence of physico-chemical carrier properties on the in vitro aerosol deposition from interactive mixtures." *International Journal of Pharmaceutics* 252 (1-2):87-98. doi: 10.1016/S0378-5173(02)00621-X.

Maltz, David S., and Stephen J. Paboojian. 2011. "Device engineering insights into TOBI Podhaler: a development case study of high efficient powder delivery to cystic fibrosis patients." *Proceedings of RDD Europe*:55-65.

Olsson, Bo, and Lars Asking. 1994. "A model for the effect of inhalation device flow resistance on the peak inspiratory flow rate and its application in pharmaceutical testing." *Journal of Aerosol Medicine* 7 (2):201-204.

Ruzycki, Conor A, Emadeddin Javaheri, and Warren H Finlay. 2013. "The use of computational fluid dynamics in inhaler design." *Expert Opinion on Drug Delivery* 10 (3):307-323.

Schuster, Antje, Cynthia Haliburn, Gerd Döring, Martin Harris Goldman, and Freedom Study Group. 2013. "Safety, efficacy and convenience of colistimethate sodium dry powder for inhalation (Colobreathe DPI) in patients with cystic fibrosis: a randomised study." *Thorax* 68 (4):344-350.

Shur, Jagdeep, Sau Lee, Wallace Adams, Robert Lionberger, James Tibbatts, and Robert Price. 2012. "Effect of device design on the in vitro performance and comparability for capsule-based dry powder inhalers." *The AAPS Journal* 14 (4):667-676.

Sim, Sally, Kenneth Margo, Jonathan Parks, Ruth Howell, Gerald A Hebbink, Laurence Orlando, Ian Larson, Philip Leslie, Louise Ho, and David AV Morton. 2014. "An insight into powder entrainment and drug delivery mechanisms from a modified Rotahaler®." *International Journal of Pharmaceutics* 477 (1):351-360.

Son, Yoen-Ju, P Worth Longest, and Michael Hindle. 2012. "Aerosolization characteristics of dry powder inhaler formulations for the enhanced excipient growth application: effect of DPI design." *Respiratory Drug Delivery* 3:899-902.

Srichana, Teerapol, Gary P. Martin, and Christopher M. Marriott. 1998. "Dry powder inhalers: the influence of device resistance and powder formulation on drug and lactose deposition in vitro." *European Journal of Pharmaceutical Sciences* 7 (1):73-80.

Suwandecha, Tan, Wibul Wongpoowarak, Kittinan Maliwan, and Teerapol Srichana. 2014. "Effect of turbulent kinetic energy on dry powder inhaler performance." *Powder Technology* 267:381-391. doi: 10.1016/j.powtec.2014.07.044.

Suwandecha, Tan, Wibul Wongpoowarak, and Teerapol Srichana. 2016. "Computer-aided design of dry powder inhalers using computational fluid dynamics to assess performance." *Pharmaceutical Development and Technology* 21 (1):54-60. doi: 10.3109/10837450.2014.965325.

Tang, Patricia, Hak-Kim Chan, Dorrilyn Rajbhandari, and Paul Phipps. 2011. "Method to introduce mannitol powder to intubated patients to improve sputum clearance." *Journal of Aerosol Medicine and Pulmonary Drug Delivery* 24 (1):1-9.

Tiano, Susan L, and Richard N Dalby. 1996. "Comparison of a respiratory suspension aerosolized by an air-jet and an ultrasonic nebulizer." *Pharmaceutical Development and Technology* 1 (3):261-268.

Timsina, M. P., Gary P. Martin, Christopher Marriott, David Ganderton, and Michael Yianneskis. 1994. "Drug delivery to the respiratory tract using dry powder inhalers." *International Journal of Pharmaceutics* 101 (1):1-13. doi: 10.1016/0378-5173(94)90070-1.

Tong, Zhenbo, Santoso Adi, Runyu Yang, Hak-Kim Chan, and Aibing Yu. 2011. "Numerical investigation of the de-agglomeration mechanisms of fine powders on mechanical impaction." *Journal of Aerosol Science* 42 (11):811-819.

Tong, Zhenbo, Runyu Yang, Kaiwei Chu, Aibing Yu, Santoso Adi, and Hak-Kim Chan. 2010. "Numerical study of the effects of particle size and polydispersity on the agglomerate dispersion in a cyclonic flow." *Chemical Engineering Journal* 164 (2):432-441.

Van Der Palen, Job, Michiel M Eijsvogel, Bart F Kuipers, Maria Schipper, and Niek A Vermue. 2007. "Comparison of the Diskus® Inhaler and the Handihaler® regarding preference and ease of use." *Journal of Aerosol Medicine* 20 (1):38-44.

Voshaar, Thomas, Monica Spinola, Patrick Linnane, Alice Campanini, Daniel Lock, Anthony Lafratta, Mario Scuri, Barbara Ronca, and Andrea S Melani. 2014. "Comparing usability of NEXThaler® with other inhaled corticosteroid/long-acting β2-agonist fixed combination dry powder inhalers in asthma patients." *Journal of Aerosol Medicine and Pulmonary Drug Delivery* 27 (5):363-370.

Wong, William, David F Fletcher, Daniela Traini, Hak-Kim Chan, and Paul M Young. 2012. "The use of computational approaches in inhaler development." *Advanced Drug Delivery Reviews* 64 (4):312-322.

Zhou, Qi, Patricia Tang, Sharon Shui Yee Leung, John Gar Yan Chan, and Hak-Kim Chan. 2014. "Emerging inhalation aerosol devices and strategies: Where are we headed?" *Advanced Drug Delivery Reviews* 75:3-17. doi: 10.1016/j.addr.2014.03.006.

Chapter 7

In Vitro Quality Control of Dry Powder Inhaler

7.1. Introduction

This chapter contains information on the *in vitro* quality control of dry powder inhalers. Most of the information has been abstracted from the British Pharmacopeia (BP), United States Pharmacopeia (USP), European Pharmacopeia (EP) and European Medicines Agency (EMA). Some examples of the quality control data have been provided.

Dry powders for inhalers are intended for lung administration in order to obtain a local or systemic effect (Figure 7.1). They contain one or more active substances that are dispersed in a suitable vehicle. Preparations of the dry powder for inhalation may contain diluents. These diluents do not adversely affect the functions of the mucosa in the respiratory tract. Preparations for inhalation are supplied in multidose or single-dose containers.

The size of aerosol particles to be inhaled is precisely controlled so that a significant fraction is deposited in the deep lung. The fine-particle characteristics of DPIs are determined by the method for aerodynamic assessment of fine particles.

In assessing the uniformity of a delivered dose of a multidose inhaler, it is not sufficient to test a single inhaler. Manufacturers must substitute procedures which take inter- and intra-inhaler dose uniformity into account. A suitable procedure based on the intra-inhaler test would be to collect each of the specified doses at the beginning, middle and end of the number of doses stated on the label from separate inhalers.

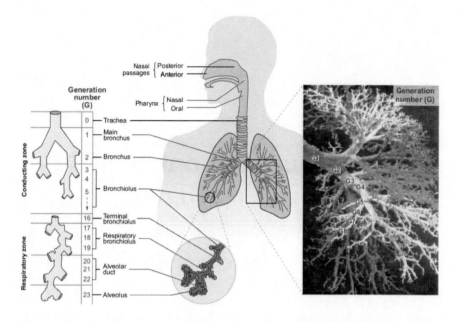

Figure 7.1. Airway generation and sizes from the trachea to alveoli. (Reprinted from Kleinstreuer, C. et al., Annual Review of Biomedical Engineering, 10, 195-220, 2008. With permission from Annual Reviews)

7.2. Labeling

For the metered-dose preparations, the delivered dose must be stated on the label: except for preparations for which the dose has been established as a predispensed-dose and minimum recommended dose.

The dry powder for an inhaler is presented as either single-dose powder inhalers or as multidose powder inhalers. To facilitate their use, additional active substances may be combined with a suitable carrier. For pre-metered inhalers, the inhaler is loaded with powders pre-dispensed in capsules or other suitable pharmaceutical forms. For inhalers using a powder reservoir, the dose is created by a metering mechanism within the inhaler. The delivered dose is the dose delivered from the inhaler. For some preparations, the dose has been established as a metered dose or as a premetered dose. The metered dose is calculated from the delivered dose plus the amount deposited on the inhaler.

7.3. Uniformity of the Delivered Dose

The dose collection apparatus must be capable of quantitatively capturing the delivered dose. A dose collection apparatus may be connected to a flow system according to the scheme specified in Figure 7.2. The dimensions of the tube and filter should accommodate the measured flow rate unless otherwise stated. For determination of the test flow rate and duration using the dose collection tube, an associated flow system, a suitable differential pressure meter and a suitable flow meter calibrated for the flow leaving the meter are required according to the following procedure.

Prepare the inhaler for use and connect it to the inlet of the apparatus using a mouthpiece adapter to ensure an airtight seal. Connect one port of a differential pressure meter to the pressure reading point, P1 (Figure 7.2) and let the other to be open to the atmosphere. Switch on the pump, open the 2-way solenoid valve and adjust the flow control valve until the pressure drop across the inhaler is 4.0 kPa (40.8 cm H_2O) as indicated by the differential pressure meter. Remove the inhaler from the mouthpiece adapter without touching the flow control valve, connect a flowmeter to the inlet of the sampling apparatus. Use a flowmeter calibrated for the flow leaving the meter or calculate the volumetric flow leaving the meter (Q_{out}) using the ideal gas law. For a meter calibrated for the entering volumetric flow (Q_{in}), use the following equation:

$$Q_{out} = \frac{Q_{in} \times P_0}{P_0 - \Delta P} \tag{7.1}$$

Where,

P_0 = atmospheric pressure

ΔP = pressure drop over the meter.

Select a single inhaler and follow the labeled instructions for loading with powder into the device. Collect a total of 10 doses, three doses at the beginning, four in the middle (n/2) − 1 to (n/2) + 2, where n is the number of minimum recommended doses on the label], and three at the end, of the labeled contents following the labeled instructions. Prior to collecting each of the doses to be analyzed, clean the inhaler as directed in the labeling.

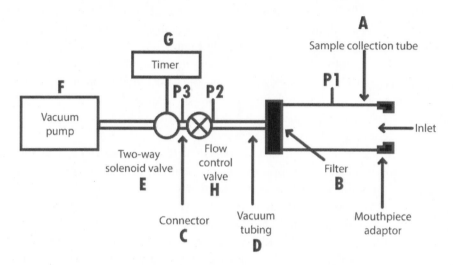

Figure 7.2. Apparatus suitable for measuring the uniformity of delivered dose of DPI. (Redrawn from British Pharmacopoeia, 2010).

For preparations containing more than one active substance, carry out the test for the uniformity of the delivered dose of each active substance. The preparation complies with the test if 9 out of 10 results lie between 75% and 125% of the average value and all lie between 65% and 135%. If 2 or 3 values lie outside the limits of 75% to 125%, repeat the test for 2 more inhalers. It is acceptable when not more than 3 of the 30 values lie outside the limits of 75% to 125%, and no value lies outside the limits of 65% to 135%.

In justified and authorized cases, these ranges may be extended, but no value should be greater than 150 % or less than 50 % of the average value.

7.4. Fine Particle Dose

Using the apparatus and procedure described in *Aerodynamic assessment of fine particles (Apparatus C, D or E)*, calculate the fine particle dose. Fine particle mass is the amount of drug that is expected to reach the lower airways obtained from the multistage impactor or any other instrument that has been calibrated (USP 35-NF 30, BP 2010). The size of the fine particle is less than 5 μm. Sometimes it is also reported as a fine particle fraction that is a fraction of fine particle mass over the total dose delivery.

7.5. Number of Deliveries per Inhaler for Multidose Inhalers

Check constant discharge doses from the inhaler until empty at the predetermined flow rate. Record the deliveries discharged. The total number of doses delivered should not be less than the number stated on the label (this test may be combined with the test for the uniformity of the delivered dose).

7.6. Aerodynamic Assessment of Fine Particles

This test is used to determine the fine particle characteristics of the aerosol clouds generated by preparations for inhalation unless otherwise justified and authorized (BP 2010) using one of the following apparatuses and test procedures. *Stage mensuration* is performed periodically together with confirmation of other dimensions critical to the effective operation of the impactor.

Re-entrainment (for apparatus D and E). To ensure efficient particle capture, each plate is coated with glycerol, silicone oil or a similar high viscosity liquid, typically deposited from a volatile solvent. Although plate coating is essential for validation of the method, it may be omitted where justified and authorized.

Mass balance. The total mass of the active substance is not less than 75% and not more than 125% of the average delivered dose determined during testing for uniformity of a delivered dose. This is not a test of the inhaler, but it serves to ensure that the results are valid.

7.6.1. Apparatus A - Glass Impinger

The glass impinger is a two stage impinger, where stage 1 is the upper impingement chamber and stage 2 is the lower impingement chamber. This apparatus is used to determine the fine particle characteristics of the aerosol clouds generated by preparations for inhalation (Figure 7.3).

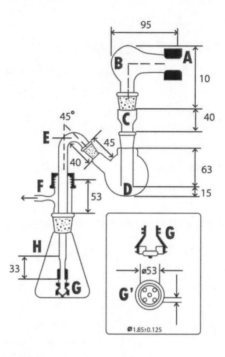

Figure 7.3. Apparatus A: glass impinger (Dimensions in millimeters; tolerances ±1 mm unless otherwise described).

Procedure for Powder Inhalers

Introduce 7 mL and 30 mL of a suitable solvent into the upper and lower impingement chambers, respectively. Connect all the components. Ensure that the assembly is vertical and adequately supported and the jet-spacer peg of the lower jet assembly just touches the bottom of the lower impingement chamber. Without the inhaler in place, connect a suitable pump to the outlet of the apparatus. Adjust the air flow through the apparatus, as measured at the inlet to the throat, to 60 ± 5 LPM. Prepare the inhaler for use and locate the mouthpiece in the apparatus using a suitable adapter. Switch on the pump for 5 s. Switch off the pump and remove the inhaler. Repeat the discharge sequence. The number of discharges should be minimized and typically would not be greater than 10.

Dismantle the apparatus. Wash the inner surface of the inlet tube to the lower impingement chamber and its outer surface that projects into the chamber with a suitable solvent. Collect the washings in the lower impingement chamber. Determine the content of active substance in this solution. Calculate the amount of active substance collected in the lower impingement chamber per discharge and express the results as a percentage of the dose stated on the label.

7.6.2. Apparatus C - Multi-Stage Liquid Impinger

Fine Particle Dose and Particle Size Distribution

The multi-stage liquid impinger consists of impaction stages 1 (pre-separator), 2, 3 and 4 and an integral filter stage (stage 5) (Figure 7.4). An impaction stage comprises an upper horizontal metal partition wall through which a metal inlet jet tube with its impaction plate is protruding. A glass cylinder with sampling port forms the vertical wall of the stage and a lower horizontal metal partition wall through which the tube connects to the next lower stage. The tube into stage 4 ends in a multi-jet arrangement. The impaction plate is secured in a metal frame that is fastened by 2 wires to a sleeve secured on the jet tube. The horizontal face of the collection plate is perpendicular to the axis of the jet tube and centrally aligned. The upper surface of the impaction plate is slightly raised above the edge of the metal frame. A recess around the perimeter of the horizontal partition wall guides the position of the glass cylinder. The glass cylinders are sealed against the horizontal partition walls with gaskets and clamped together by 6 bolts. The sampling ports are sealed by stoppers. The bottom-side of the lower partition wall of stage 4 has a concentrical protrusion fitted with a rubber O-ring which seals against the edge of a filter placed in the filter holder. The filter holder is constructed as a basin with a concentrical recess in which a perforated filter support is flush-fitted. The filter holder consists of 76 mm diameter filters. The assembly of the impaction stages is clamped onto the filter holder by 2 snap-locks. Connect an induction port (Figure 7.5) onto the stage 1 inlet jet tube of the impinger. A rubber O-ring on the jet tube provides an airtight connection to the induction port. A suitable mouthpiece adapter is used to provide an airtight seal between the inhaler and the induction port.

Procedure for Powder Inhalers

Place a suitable low resistance filter capable of quantitatively collecting the active substance in stage 5 and assemble the apparatus. Connect the apparatus to a flow system according to the scheme specified in Figure 7.6.

Unless otherwise defined, conduct the test at the flow rate, Q_{out}, used in the test for determination of the uniformity of delivered dose, drawing 4 L of air from the mouthpiece of the inhaler and through the apparatus. Connect a flowmeter to the induction port. Use a flowmeter calibrated for the volumetric flow leaving the meter or calculate the volumetric flow leaving the meter (Q_{out}) using the ideal gas law.

Adjust the flow control valve to achieve a steady flow through the system at the required rate, Q_{out} (±5%). Switch off the pump and ensure that the critical flow occurs in the flow control valve by the following procedure. With the inhaler in place and the test flow rate established, measure the absolute pressure on both sides of the control valve (pressure reading points P2 and P3 in Figure 7.6). A ratio P3/P2 of less than or equal to 0.5 indicates a critical flow. Switch to a more powerful pump and re-measure the test flow rate if a critical flow is not indicated. Dispense 20 mL of a solvent, capable of dissolving the active substance into each of the 4 upper stages of the apparatus and replace the stoppers. Tilt the apparatus to wet the stoppers, thereby neutralizing the electrostatic charge. Place a suitable mouthpiece adapter in position at the end of the induction port.

Prepare the powder inhaler for use according to the patient instructions. With the pump running and the 2-way solenoid valve closed, locate the mouthpiece of the inhaler in the mouthpiece adapter. Discharge the powder into the apparatus by opening the valve for the required time, T (±5%).

Repeat the procedure. The number of discharges should be minimized and typically would not be greater than 10. The number of discharges is sufficient to ensure an accurate and precise determination of fine particle dose. Dismantle the filter stage of the apparatus. Carefully remove the filter and extract the active substance into an aliquot of solvent. Remove the induction port and mouthpiece adapter from the apparatus and extract the active substance into an aliquot of solvent. If necessary, rinse the inside of the inlet jet tube to stage 1 with solvent, allowing the solvent to flow into the stage. Extract the active substance from the inner walls and the collection plate for each of the 4 upper stages of the apparatus into the solution in the respective stage by carefully tilting and rotating the apparatus, carefully observing that no liquid transfer occurs between the stages. Using a suitable method of analysis, determine the amount of active substance present in each of the aliquots of solvent.

Calculate the fine particle dose (see Calculations).

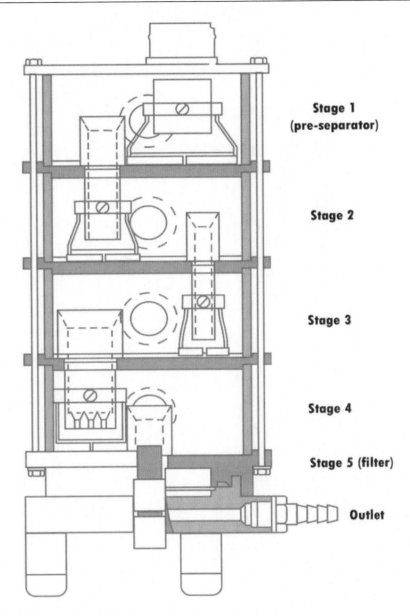

Figure 7.4. Apparatus C: multi-stage liquid impinger. (Adapted from USP35–NF30, United States Pharmacopeial Convention, 2010).

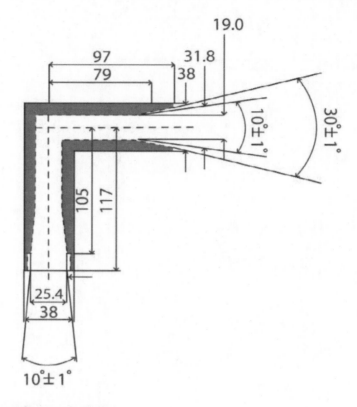

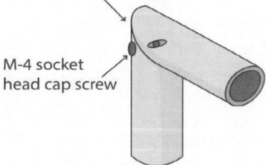

Joint must be leak tight

M-4 socket
head cap screw

Figure 7.5. Induction port. Dimensions in millimeters unless otherwise stated. (Adapted from British Pharmacopoeia, 2010).

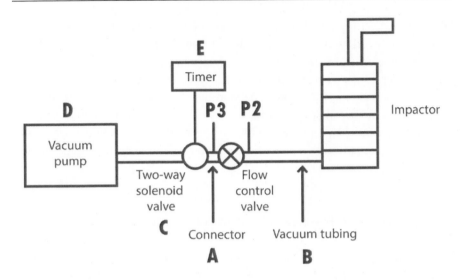

Figure 7.6. Experimental set up for testing dry powder inhalers. (Adapted from British Pharmacopoeia, 2010).

7.6.3. Apparatus D - Andersen Cascade Impactor

The Andersen cascade impactor consists of 8 stages together with a final filter. The material of construction may be aluminum, stainless steel or other suitable material. The stages are clamped together and sealed with O-rings. Critical dimensions are applied by the manufacturer of the apparatus D. In use, some occlusion and wear of the holes will occur. In-use mensuration tolerances need to be justified. The entry cone of the impactor is connected to an induction port (Figure 7.7). A suitable mouthpiece adapter is used to provide an airtight seal between the inhaler and the induction port. In the configuration for powder inhalers, a pre-separator is placed above the top stage to collect large masses of non-respirable powder. To accommodate high flow rates through the impactor, the outlet nipple, used to connect the impactor to the vacuum system, is enlarged to have an internal diameter of greater than or equal to 8 mm.

Procedure for Powder Inhalers

The aerodynamic cut-off diameters of the individual stages of this apparatus are currently not well-established at flow rates other than 28.3 LPM.

Users must justify and validate the use of the impactor in the chosen conditions when flow rates that are different from 28.3 LPM are selected.

Assemble the Andersen cascade impactor with the pre-separator and a suitable filter in place and ensure that the system is airtight. Depending on the product characteristics, the pre-separator may be omitted where justified. Stages 6 and 7 may also be omitted at high flow rates if justified. The pre-separator may be coated in the same way as for the plates or may contain 10 mL of a suitable solvent. Connect the apparatus to a flow system according to the scheme specified in Figure 7.6.

7.6.4. Apparatus E - Next Generation Impactor

Apparatus E is a cascade impactor with 7 stages and a micro-orifice collector (MOC). Over the flow rate range of 30 LPM to 100 LPM, the 50 percent efficiency cut-off diameters (D_{50} values) that range between 0.24 μm to 11.7 μm will be evenly spaced on a logarithmic scale. In this flow range, there are always at least 5 stages with D_{50} values between 0.5 μm and 6.5 μm. The collection efficiency curves for each stage are sharp and minimize overlap between stages.

The material of construction may be aluminum, stainless steel or other suitable material. The configuration of the impactor has removable impaction cups with all the cups in one plane (Figure 7.8). There are 3 main sections to the impactor; the bottom frame that holds the impaction cups, the sealed body that holds the jets and the lid that contains the interstage passage ways. Multiple nozzles are used except at the first stage (Figure 7.9). The flow passes through the impactor in a saw-tooth pattern.

In routine operation, the sealed body and lid are held together as a single assembly. The impaction cups are accessible when this assembly is opened at the end of an inhaler test. The cups are held in a support tray so that all cups can be removed from the impactor simultaneously by lifting the tray. An induction port with internal dimensions (relevant to the airflow path), defined in Figure 7.7, connects to the impactor inlet. A pre-separator can be added when required, typically with powder inhalers and its connections between the induction port and the impactor. A suitable mouthpiece adapter is used to provide an airtight seal between the inhaler and the induction port.

Apparatus E contains a terminal Micro-Orifice Collector (MOC) that for most formulations will eliminate the need for a final filter as determined by the method validation. The MOC is an impactor plate with nominally 4032 holes, each approximately 70 μm in diameter. Most particles that are not captured on stage 7 of the impactor will be captured on the cup surface below the MOC. For impactors operated at 60 LPM, the MOC is capable of collecting 80% of 0.14 μm particles. For formulations with a significant fraction of particles not captured by the MOC, there is an optional filter holder that can replace the MOC or be placed downstream of the MOC (a glass fiber filter is suitable).

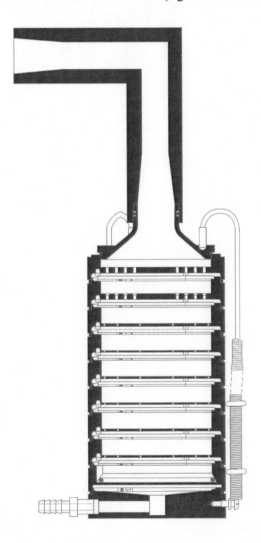

Figure 7.7. Apparatus D: *Andersen cascade impactor used for* DPI. (Adapted from British Pharmacopoeia, 2010).

Procedure for Powder Inhalers

Assemble the apparatus with the pre-separator. Depending on the product characteristics, the pre-separator may be omitted where justified. Place cups into the apertures in the cup tray. Insert the cup tray into the bottom frame and lower into place. Close the impactor lid with the sealed body attached and operate the handle to lock the impactor together so that the system is airtight.

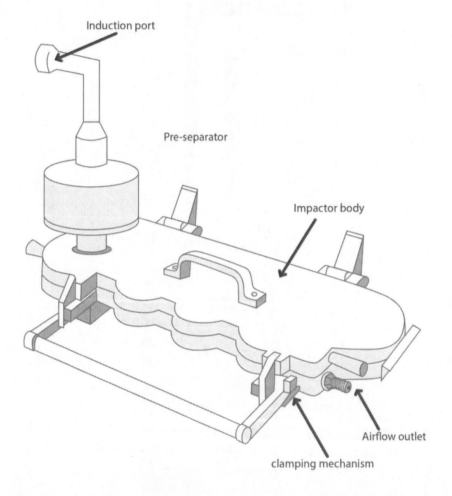

Figure 7.8. Apparatus E shown with the pre-separator in place. (Adapted from British Pharmacopoeia, 2010).

When a pre-separator is used, it should be assembled as follows: assemble the pre-separator by inserting it into the pre-separator base. Fit the pre-separator base to the impactor inlet. Add 15 mL of solvent for sample recovery to the central cup of the pre-separator insert. Place the pre-separator body on top of this assembly and close the 2 catches.

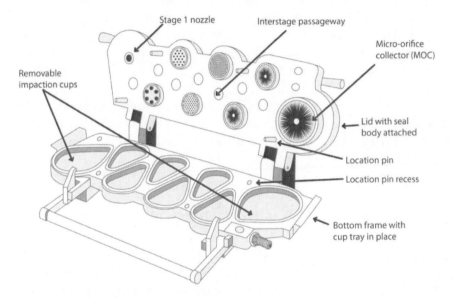

Figure 7.9. Apparatus E and its components. (Adapted from British Pharmacopoeia, 2010).

Connect an induction port that has internal dimensions defined in Figure 7.5 to the impactor inlet or pre-separator inlet. Place a suitable mouthpiece adapter in position at the end of the induction port so that the mouthpiece end of the inhaler, when inserted, lines up along the horizontal axis of the induction port. When attached to the mouthpiece adapter, the inhaler is positioned in the same orientation as intended for use. Connect the apparatus to a flow system according to the scheme specified in Figure 7.8.

Prepare the powder inhaler according to the instructions to the patient. With the pump running and the 2-way solenoid valve closed, locate the mouthpiece of the inhaler into the mouthpiece adapter. Discharge the powder into the apparatus by opening the valve for the required time, T (± 5%).

Repeat the discharge sequence. The number of discharges should be minimized and typically would not be greater than 10. The number of discharges is sufficient to ensure an accurate and precise determination of fine particle dose.

Dismantle the apparatus and recover the active substance as follows: remove the induction port and mouthpiece adapter from the pre-separator, when used, and recover the deposited active substance into an aliquot of solvent. When used, remove the pre-separator from the impactor, being careful to avoid spilling the cup liquid into the impactor. Recover the active substance from the pre-separator. Open the impactor by releasing the handle and lifting the lid.

Remove the cup tray along with the collection cups and recover the active substance in each cup into an aliquot of solvent. Using a suitable method of analysis, determine the quantity of active substance present in each of the solvent aliquots.

7.7. Calculations

From the analysis of the solutions, calculate the mass of the active substance deposited on each stage per discharge and the mass of the active substance per discharge deposited in the induction port, mouthpiece adapter and when used, the pre-separator.

Starting at the final collection site (filter or MOC), derive a table of cumulative mass versus the cut-off diameter of the respective stage. Calculate by interpolation the mass of the active substance less than 5 μm. This is the Fine Particle Dose (FPD).

If necessary and where appropriate (e.g., where there is a log-normal distribution), plot the cumulative fraction of the active substance versus cut-off the diameter on a log probability paper and use this plot to determine the values for the Mass Median Aerodynamic Diameter (MMAD) and Geometric Standard Deviation (GSD) as appropriate (as detailed in Chapter 1). Appropriate computational methods may also be used.

7.8. Other Quality Control of Finished Products of Dry Powder Inhaler

The products have to be controlled in all batches as follows.

7.8.1. Moisture Content

Moisture control is specified in the finished products. It is important because it is one parameter to be controlled assure that the product is stable over its shelf life.

7.8.2. Microbiological Limits

The microbial limit is specified in the specific monograph.

7.8.3. Simulated Patient Use

The simulation of patient use of an inhaler through the device should be carried out to obtain the data close to real life use. The patient parameters such as flow rate, inhalation volume and environmental aspects should mimic real life as close as possible to obtain realizable data. Therefore, the simulated *in vitro* system should be close to the *in vivo* as much as possible.

7.8.4. Reusable vs Disposable Reliability Testing

The quality control of the dry powder inhaler usually consists of assay, delivered dose, dose uniformity, content uniformity and fine particle fraction. Other quality controls are also necessary such as moisture content, microbial limit and number per container (Table 7.1).

The following tests are applicable to metered-dose inhalers that are formulated as suspensions or solutions of active drug in propellants and dry powder inhalers presented as single or multidose units. The following test methods are specific to the aforementioned inhalers and may require modification when testing alternative inhalation technologies (e.g., breath-actuated metered-dose inhalers or dose-metering nebulizers). However, Pharmacopeial requirements for all dose-metering inhalation dosage forms require determination of the delivered dose and aerodynamic size distribution. In all cases, and for all tests, prepare and test the inhaler as directed on the label and the instructions for use.

**Table 7.1. Dry powder inhaler quality control
(Adapted from EMA Guideline on the pharmaceutical
quality of inhalation and nasal products, 2006)**

Drug Product Specification	Device metered	Pre-metered
(a) Description	Yes	Yes
(b) Assay	Yes	Yes
(c) Moisture content	Yes	Yes
(d) Mean delivered dose	Yes	Yes
(e) Delivered dose uniformity	Yes	Yes
(f) Content uniformity	No	No
(g) Fine particle mass	Yes	Yes
(h) Microbial limit	Yes	Yes
(i) Number per container	Yes	No

An example of a quality control report of two products based on an evaluation of MMAD, GSD, FPF and emitted dose (Table 7.2).

Table 7.2. Quality control of two dry powder inhalers (mean ± sd, n= 10)

Items	Product A	Product B
MMAD (μm)	3.5±0.1	2.1±0.1
GSD	1.9±0.0	1.7±0.0
FPM (μg)	8.9±0.7	10.5±0.6
Emitted dose (μg)	23.5±0.6	20.1±0.6

The MMADs of product A and product B are significantly different ($P<0.01$), where the GSDs of the two products are very similar. The FPM and emitted dose showed trivial differences. It can be explained that the lung deposition is expected to be different because the MMAD is different resulting in different depositions in the airway. The smaller MMAD is expected to penetrate deeper in the lung.

References

BP 2010. 2010. *British Pharmacopoeia*. London, UK: The Stationery Office Ltd.

EMEA. 2006. Guideline on the pharmaceutical quality of inhalation and nasal products.

Kleinstreuer, Clement, Zhe Zhang, and James F. Donohue. 2008. "Targeted drug-aerosol delivery in the human respiratory system." *Annual Review of Biomedical Engineering* 10:195-220.

Ph. Eur. 8th Edition. 2016. "Preparations for Inhalation: Aerodynamic Assessment of Fine Particles." In *European Pharmacopoeia* Strasbourg, France: Council of Europe.

USP 35-NF 30. 2010. *United States Pharmacopeia and National Formulary (USP35–NF30)*. Vol. 2, *United States Pharmacopeia—National Formulary*. Rockville, MD: United States Pharmacopeial Convention.

About the Author

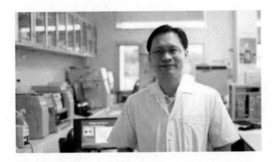

Dr. Teerapol Srichana graduated from Prince of Songkla University in 1989 (Bachelor of Pharmacy), hold a Master of Pharmaceutical Science from the Gent University, Belgium, and a Ph.D. from the King's College London, United Kingdom in 1998. Currently he is an Associate Professor in the Department of Pharmaceutical Technology, Prince of Songkla University (PSU), Thailand and also serves as the Dean of the Graduate School at the PSU. He is currently the Director of Drug Delivery System Excellence Center and NANOTEC-PSU Center of Excellence on Drug Delivery. In his scientific career, he has served on numerous academic boards and committees, and published more than 150 research articles, reviews and book chapters, which are highly cited.

Index

T

U

V

W